CONQUER NEUROPATHY: THE POWER OF THE R.E.S.T.O.R.E. METHOD

Dr. Omar Clark D.C.
Conquer Neuropathy: The Power of the R.E.S.T.O.R.E. Method

Published by Spines
ISBN:979-8-89569-955-3

CONQUER NEUROPATHY: THE POWER OF THE R.E.S.T.O.R.E. METHOD

DR. OMAR CLARK, D.C.

GET ACCESS TO YOUR
FREE NEUROPATHY RELIEF
GIFTS BELOW

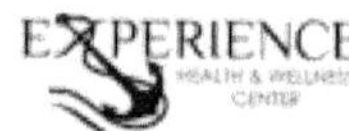
EXPERIENCE
HEALTH & WELLNESS
CENTER

- Neuropathy Health Journal
- Relieving Neuropathy Guide
- 25 Anti-Inflammatory Recipes
- Nerve Damage Quiz
- Free Health Masterclass
- 30-Day Nutrition Plan
- Neuropathy Relief Handbook

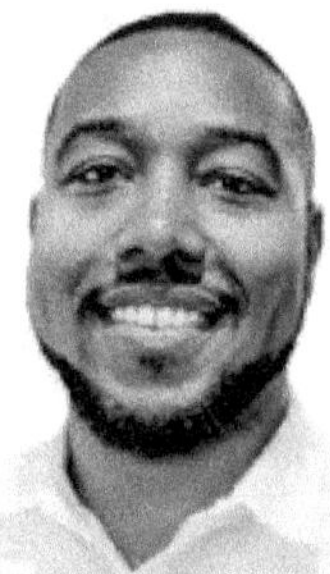
EXPERIENCE

SCAN ME DR. OMAR CLARK DC

CONTENTS

FOREWORD

Neuropathy, a relentless adversary in the world of chronic pain, can make those affected feel trapped, isolated, and drained of their quality of life. But even in the darkest times, hope can shine through, proving that healing is possible with innovative solutions.

Enter Dr. Omar Clark, D.C., a visionary in the field and a cherished member of the Driven Doc community at The Data Driven Practice. Dr. Clark has dedicated his career to untangling the complexities of neuropathy, helping patients reclaim their lives. His groundbreaking R.E.S.T.O.R.E Method, detailed in his transformative new book, offers a beacon of hope for those who have long sought relief.

As a fellow chiropractor and passionate advocate for neuropathy sufferers, I've witnessed firsthand the remarkable impact of Dr. Clark's approach. His unwavering commitment to patient care, deep empathy, and relentless pursuit of knowledge have touched countless lives, inspiring hope and fostering healing.

"Conquer Neuropathy: The Power of the R.E.S.T.O.R.E. Method" is more than just a book; it's a testament to the resilience of the human spirit, a roadmap to recovery, and a celebration of the transformative power of integrative care. Dr. Clark's holistic approach, refined over years of clinical practice, targets the root causes of neuropathy, offering a comprehensive and sustainable solution.

But this book is also a story of partnership and dedication. It's a tribute to the unwavering support of Dr. Clark's wife, Jazmin, and their dedicated team at Experience Health & Wellness Center - Cape Coral's premier chiropractic center. Together, they've created a haven of healing where patients are empowered to take control of their health and embark on a journey toward pain-free living.

Within these pages, you'll find a wealth of knowledge, practical tools, and a renewed sense of hope. The R.E.S.T.O.R.E Method is your guide, Dr. Clark is your ally, and a brighter future awaits. Embrace this transformative journey and reclaim your life from the clutches of neuropathy.

xiii

Dr. Cory Frogley, D.C.
The Data Driven Practice

DISCLAIMER

The information provided in this book is intended for educational purposes only and is not a substitute for professional medical advice. The author and publisher are not liable for any adverse effects or consequences resulting from the use of the information presented herein. Always consult your physician or a qualified healthcare provider regarding any health concerns or before making any decisions related to your health or treatment.

The patient or any other person responsible for payment has the right to refuse to pay, cancel payment, or request a refund for any service, examination, or treatment performed as a result of and within 72 hours of responding to this advertisement for free, discounted, or reduced-fee services. All services, including any offered X-rays or exams, will only be provided if deemed medically necessary. Dr. Omar Clark, Doctor of Chiropractic (D.C.), licensed in the state of Florida.

ABOUT THE AUTHOR

Hi, I'm Dr. Omar Clark, D.C., a chiropractor, and the founder of the RESTORE Neuropathy Program and the Experience Health & Wellness Center in Cape Coral, Florida - a chiropractic center dedicated to your well-being. I'm also the author of this book, Conquer Neuropathy: The Power of the R.E.S.T.O.R.E. Method.

In this book, I will share with you my personal journey of discovering the truth about how to significantly improve neuropathy naturally and how I developed a comprehensive program that has helped thousands of people regain their health and happiness.

It all started with a patient named Samantha, who came to me with chronic spinal pain. As I examined her, I found out that she had been suffering from neuropathy for years without any effective treatment or relief. She had almost given up hope. And I could see the frustration in her eyes.

As a dedicated healthcare professional, I couldn't accept that. I made a promise to myself that day to find a solution for her neuropathy, to restore her hope, and to help her regain control of her life.

And so, I immersed myself in the latest research, attended conferences, and collaborated with other practitioners who shared my passion for finding natural solutions. I was determined to uncover the truth about how to effectively treat neuropathy and help my patients reclaim their lives.

Months turned into years, and my dedication never wavered. I tested different techniques, explored alternative therapies, and fine-tuned my understanding of this complex condition. I witnessed firsthand the power of combining holistic approaches, cutting-edge technology, and personalized care.

Through this relentless effort, I finally developed a comprehensive program, the RESTORE Neuropathy Program, that addresses the root causes of neuropathy and provides a pathway to recovery.

But my journey didn't stop with Samantha. I realized that there were thousands of individuals out there suffering silently from neuropathy, just like she had been for years. That's when I knew I had to share my knowledge and breakthrough discoveries with the world.

That's why I wrote this book - to empower you with a deeper understanding of neuropathy, its causes, and how you can effectively manage it naturally using the R.E.S.T.O.R.E. Method.

You will also hear from some of my patients who have successfully completed the RESTORE neuropathy program and how it improved their lives. And I want you to be one of them.

That's why I invite you to take action today and join me on this journey of reversing neuropathy naturally.

Don't let neuropathy rob you of your joy and freedom. Don't let it stop you from living the life you deserve.

You have the power to heal yourself. You have the power to restore your health and happiness.

All you need is the right guidance, the right support, and the right program.

And that's what I'm here to offer you.

So don't wait any longer. Visit our website, efchealth. com/neuropathy/, and contact us today to get started on the RESTORE neuropathy program.

We look forward to hearing from you soon and helping you relieve your neuropathy naturally.

A little more about me:

I received my B.S. in Health Promotions at Liberty University as a collegiate athlete. From there, I pursued a Master's in Health and Wellness. I am also board-certified in neuropathy. I always had a passion for true health and assisting others in becoming educated on what true health and healing are.

I met my wife, Jazmin, in college and have been married for over ten years; we have three amazing little blessings. Having children has opened my eyes to the significance of educating families on the importance of chiropractic care starting as a newborn. I also gained clinical experience in pediatric and maternal chiropractic care, which deepened my passion for serving families.

With my fun, loving, passionate, caring spirit, I am committed to serving the beautiful Cape Coral community and leading you and your families to experience what it means to live a life of optimal health.

Experience Health & Wellness Center, your Cape Coral chiropractic center, is committed to building a healthy community one family at a time.

NEUROPATHY UNVEILED: A CLOSER LOOK

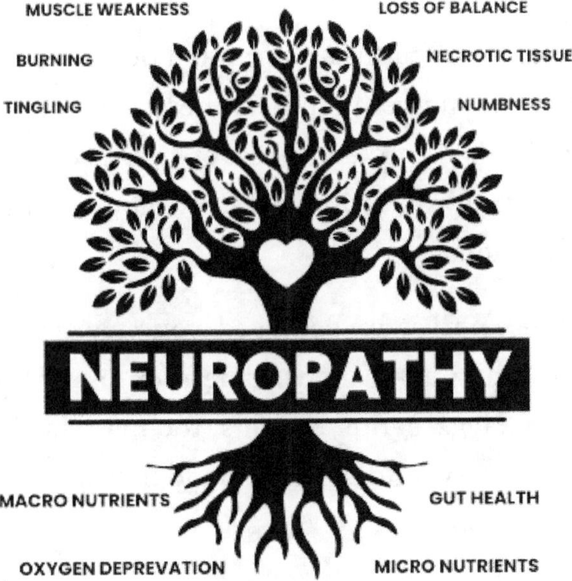

Imagine waking up one day unable to feel the ground beneath your feet. For millions living with peripheral neuropathy, this is more than a fear—it's reality. Welcome to *Conquer Neuropathy: The Power of the R.E.S.T.O.R.E. Method*. I'm going to dive into the problem of neuropathy, uncovering its causes, progression, and profound effects on daily life. With real stories of resilience and practical advice, equipping you with the tools to detect and address neuropathy early—and take back control of your health.

Understanding Peripheral Neuropathy

Peripheral neuropathy is a term that describes damage to the nerves that carry messages from your brain and spinal cord to the rest of your body. These nerves control your movements, sensations, and organ functions.

When these nerves are damaged, you may experience numbness, tingling, pain, weakness, or loss of balance in your feet, legs, hands, or arms. You may also have problems with your digestion, bladder, heart, or sexual function.

What Causes Neuropathy?

There are many different causes of neuropathy. Let's discuss some of the most common causes.

Diabetes

Diabetes is a chronic condition that affects how your body regulates blood sugar (glucose). When blood sugar levels become chronically elevated, it can damage various organs and tissues, including your nerves. This nerve damage is a major contributor to neuropathy.

Here's a breakdown of the main types of diabetes:

- **Type 1 Diabetes:** This autoimmune disease occurs when your body attacks the cells in your pancreas that produce insulin. Insulin is a hormone crucial for unlocking your cells and allowing them to absorb sugar from the bloodstream. Without enough insulin, sugar builds up in the blood, leading to the hallmark symptoms of diabetes.
- **Type 2 Diabetes:** This is the most common form of diabetes. In type 2 diabetes, your body either develops resistance to insulin's effects, or it doesn't produce enough insulin. This also leads to high blood sugar levels.

- **Gestational Diabetes:** This form of diabetes develops during pregnancy and usually resolves after childbirth. However, it can increase your risk of developing type 2 diabetes later in life.

If you're concerned about your risk of diabetes or neuropathy, a crucial first step is to check your blood sugar levels. Early detection and management of diabetes are essential to prevent complications like nerve damage. Here's how you can get started:

- **Talk to your doctor:** Discuss your risk factors and symptoms. They can advise you on the best approach for testing your blood sugar.
- **Consider home blood sugar monitoring:** With your doctor's guidance, you might use a glucometer, a small device that allows you to easily check your blood sugar levels at home.
- **Start with small changes:** If your blood sugar levels are elevated, even minor adjustments to your diet and lifestyle can make a significant difference.

Remember, early detection and management are key. By taking charge of your blood sugar health, you can significantly reduce your risk of complications like neuropathy. The RESTORE neuropathy program will be right here to support you every step of the way, providing resources and guidance to empower you on your journey towards optimal health.

Alcoholism

Chronic alcohol consumption is a significant risk factor for neuropathy. Alcohol damages your nerves in two main ways:

- **Direct Toxicity:** Alcohol itself is a neurotoxin, meaning it can directly damage the structure and function of your nerve cells. Imagine your nerves as delicate communication cables. Excessive alcohol acts like a poison, disrupting the signals traveling through these cables, leading to symptoms like numbness, tingling, and weakness.
- **Indirect Damage:** Alcohol disrupts the blood supply to your nerves. Think of your nerves like intricate electrical circuits. Healthy blood flow is crucial for delivering oxygen and essential nutrients to keep these circuits functioning properly. Alcohol damages the delicate lining of blood vessels, leading to restricted blood flow and depriving your nerves of the vital resources they need to

thrive. This lack of oxygen and nutrients further contributes to nerve damage.

Excessive alcohol consumption also depletes your body's B vitamins, particularly B1 (thiamine) and B12. These B vitamins play a critical role in nerve health and function. Deficiencies in these vitamins can worsen neuropathy symptoms and lead to a condition called Wernicke-Korsakoff syndrome, known for causing memory problems, balance issues, and severe nerve damage.

If you're concerned about alcohol consumption and its impact on your nerves, the good news is that there's hope. Reducing or eliminating alcohol intake can significantly improve nerve health and potentially heal some of the damage caused by alcohol.

Vitamin B12 deficiency

Vitamin B12 deficiency is a surprisingly common culprit behind neuropathy. This essential vitamin plays a critical role in maintaining the health and function of your nervous system. Here's how a B12 deficiency can contribute to nerve damage:

- **Protecting the Myelin Sheath:** Imagine your nerves as electrical wires. The myelin sheath acts like a fatty insulating layer surrounding these wires. It protects them and ensures smooth transmission of nerve signals. Vitamin B12 is crucial for the production and maintenance of this myelin sheath. When B12 levels are low, the myelin sheath becomes damaged, exposing the nerves and leaving them vulnerable to injury. This damage disrupts nerve signals, leading to symptoms like numbness, tingling, weakness, and pain.

- **B12 and Nerve Regeneration:** Beyond protection, vitamin B12 is also involved in nerve cell regeneration and repair. A deficiency can hinder your body's ability to repair damaged nerves, further worsening neuropathy symptoms.

So who's most at risk? Certain factors increase your risk of developing a B12 deficiency:

- **Diet:** Strict vegetarians and vegans are at higher risk, as B12 is naturally found in animal products like meat, poultry, fish, and eggs.
- **Age:** As we age, our ability to absorb B12 from food can decline.
- **Digestive Issues:** Conditions like Crohn's

disease or pernicious anemia can interfere with B12 absorption.

If you suspect a B12 deficiency, a doctor can perform a simple blood test to confirm it. Treatment typically involves B12 supplements, which can be taken orally or through injections.

For those who can consume animal products, incorporating these B12-rich foods into your diet can be beneficial:

- Meat, poultry, and fish
- Eggs
- Dairy products
- Fortified foods like some cereals and nutritional yeast

Remember: Always consult a doctor before starting any new supplements, especially if you have any underlying health conditions or are taking medications. The RESTORE method recognizes the importance of addressing B12 deficiency as part of our comprehensive approach to neuropathy management.

Autoimmune diseases

Autoimmune diseases are a group of conditions where your body's immune system, normally tasked with fighting off invaders like bacteria and viruses, mistakenly identifies healthy tissues as a threat. In some cases, this misplaced attack can target your nerves, leading to neuropathy. Here's a closer look at how autoimmune diseases can damage your nervous system:

- Certain autoimmune diseases, like Guillain-Barré syndrome and chronic inflammatory demyelinating polyneuropathy (CIDP), directly attack the nerves themselves. This attack can damage the myelin sheath, the protective layer surrounding nerves, or the nerves themselves. This disrupts nerve signaling, causing symptoms like weakness, numbness, tingling, and pain.
- Many autoimmune diseases involve chronic inflammation, a cellular firestorm that damages surrounding tissues. When nerves are caught in the crossfire of this inflammation, it can lead to nerve damage and neuropathy symptoms.

Examples of Autoimmune Diseases Affecting Nerves:

- **Guillain-Barré Syndrome (GBS):** A rapid onset of muscle weakness, often starting in the legs and spreading upwards, is a hallmark of GBS. This is caused by the immune system attacking the myelin sheath of peripheral nerves.

- **Chronic Inflammatory Demyelinating Polyneuropathy (CIDP):** Similar to GBS, but with a more gradual progression of weakness, numbness, and tingling.

- **Sjogren's Syndrome:** An autoimmune disease affecting the moisture-producing glands in your eyes and mouth. Some people with Sjogren's syndrome also experience neuropathy, likely due to damage to the small nerves in their hands and feet.

- **Lupus:** This systemic autoimmune disease can affect various organs, including the nervous system. Lupus-related neuropathy can cause a variety of symptoms, depending on which nerves are affected.

If you have an autoimmune disease and experience any symptoms of neuropathy, it's crucial to seek medical attention promptly. Early diagnosis and treatment of the underlying autoimmune condition can help prevent further nerve damage and improve your quality of life.

Infections

Infections caused by viruses, bacteria, and even parasites can be surprising culprits behind neuropathy. These invaders can damage nerves directly or indirectly, leading to a range of symptoms like numbness, tingling, weakness, and pain. Here's a closer look at how infections can wreak havoc on your nervous system:

- Some infections, like Lyme disease caused by bacteria and shingles caused by the varicella-zoster virus (the same virus that causes chickenpox), directly target and damage nerve tissue. In the case of shingles, the virus can travel along nerve pathways, causing the characteristic painful rash and damaging the nerves themselves.
- Many infections trigger a robust immune response, leading to widespread inflammation. While this inflammation helps fight the infection, it can also damage surrounding tissues, including nerves. This collateral damage can disrupt nerve function and contribute to neuropathy symptoms.

Common Infectious Causes of Neuropathy:

- **Lyme disease:** This tick-borne illness can cause a variety of neurological symptoms, including neuropathy. The bacteria responsible for Lyme disease can directly infiltrate nerve tissue and cause inflammation, leading to nerve damage. Early diagnosis and treatment of Lyme disease are crucial to prevent long-term nerve damage.

- **Shingles:** This painful condition, characterized by a blistering rash, can also cause neuropathy. The varicella-zoster virus can travel along nerve pathways, damaging them and causing pain, numbness, and weakness in the affected area. Even after the rash clears, post-herpetic neuralgia, a form of neuropathy, can persist for months or even years.

- **HIV/AIDS:** The human immunodeficiency virus (HIV) can damage the nervous system in various ways, including causing neuropathy. HIV can directly infect nerve cells or indirectly damage them through the inflammatory response it triggers. Early diagnosis and treatment of HIV can help

prevent or slow the progression of nerve damage.
- Other Infections: While less common, other infections like **cytomegalovirus (CMV)**, **Epstein-Barr virus (EBV)**, and some bacterial infections can also cause neuropathy.

If you suspect you might have an infection and experience symptoms of neuropathy, seeking prompt medical attention is crucial. Early diagnosis and treatment of the underlying infection can help prevent further nerve damage and improve your long-term prognosis.

Medications

Medications play a vital role in treating various health conditions, but some can damage nerves directly or indirectly, leading to symptoms like numbness, tingling, weakness, and pain. Here's a breakdown of how certain medications can contribute to neuropathy:

- Chemotherapy drugs used to fight cancer are a prime example. These powerful medications work by targeting rapidly dividing cells, unfortunately, some nerve cells can be caught in the crossfire. This damage to the nerve cells' DNA can lead to neuropathy.

- Certain antibiotics, particularly those from the class known as fluoroquinolones, can disrupt the production of myelin, the protective sheath surrounding nerves. This lack of myelin leaves the nerves vulnerable to damage and can contribute to neuropathy symptoms.

Medications that can cause neuropathy:

- **Chemotherapy drugs:** These potent drugs used to treat cancer are a well-known cause of neuropathy. The specific type of chemotherapy drug and dosage can influence the risk and severity of neuropathy.
- **Antibiotics:** While uncommon, fluoroquinolone antibiotics like Ciprofloxacin (Cipro) have been associated with neuropathy.
- **Anticonvulsants:** Medications used to control seizures, like Gabapentin and Pregabalin, can sometimes cause numbness, tingling, or weakness as a side effect. This doesn't necessarily indicate neuropathy, but

it's important to discuss these sensations with your doctor.

- **Pain medications:** Certain chronic pain medications, like Tricyclic antidepressants (TCAs) and some opioids, can cause numbness or tingling as a side effect.

Medications can be lifesavers, but it's important to weigh the benefits against potential side effects like neuropathy.

Physical injuries

Accidents happen, and sometimes those accidents can leave a lasting impact on your nervous system. Physical injuries, from car accidents and falls to sports injuries and repetitive stress, can be a significant cause of neuropathy. Here's how these injuries contribute to nerve damage:

- **Direct Nerve Compression or Laceration:** The most obvious scenario is a direct blow to a nerve. A car accident, fall, or even a deep cut can severely damage or sever a nerve, leading to immediate symptoms like numbness, weakness, and pain in the affected area.

- **Stretched or Pinched Nerves:** Even less dramatic injuries can cause neuropathy. Repetitive stress injuries, like carpal tunnel syndrome, occur when a nerve gets compressed or pinched by surrounding tissues. Over time, this compression can disrupt nerve function and lead to symptoms like tingling, numbness, and weakness.
- **Blood Vessel Damage and Starved Nerves:** Physical injuries can also damage blood vessels supplying nerves. These blood vessels deliver oxygen and essential nutrients to keep nerves healthy. If these blood vessels are damaged, the nerves become starved of these vital resources, leading to nerve dysfunction and potential neuropathy symptoms.

Here are a few examples of injuries leading to neuropathy:

- **Car accidents:** The force of a car accident can cause various injuries, including nerve damage. This can range from mild compression to complete nerve severance, depending on the severity of the accident.
- **Falls:** A fall, especially on an outstretched hand, can damage nerves in the wrist or arm.

This can lead to carpal tunnel syndrome or other types of neuropathy.

- **Sports injuries:** Repetitive stress from certain sports can compress nerves, leading to neuropathy. For example, carpal tunnel syndrome is common in athletes who grip objects repeatedly, like cyclists and weightlifters.
- **Surgery:** While surgery is often necessary, it can sometimes damage nerves during the procedure. This can lead to post-surgical neuropathy, causing numbness, pain, or weakness in the affected area.

If you experience an injury and develop symptoms like numbness, tingling, or weakness, seeking medical attention promptly is crucial. Early diagnosis and treatment of nerve damage can minimize long-term complications and improve your recovery.

Idiopathic neuropathy

Neuropathy can be like a detective story – sometimes the culprit is clear, but other times, the cause remains a puzzling mystery. Idiopathic neuropathy falls into this category. It refers to nerve damage where, despite extensive evaluation, no underlying reason can be identified. While idiopathic neuropathy is considered uncommon, it can be a significant source of frustration for those affected.

Here's a closer look at this enigmatic form of neuropathy:

- Ruling Out the Usual Suspects: Extensive testing for common causes like diabetes, vitamin deficiencies, autoimmune diseases, and infections is usually conducted. If all these come back negative, then idiopathic neuropathy becomes a possibility.
- Not a Hallmark of Rarity: While uncommon, idiopathic neuropathy isn't exceptionally rare. It affects a significant portion of neuropathy cases, making it an important piece of the neuropathy puzzle.

Even though the exact cause of idiopathic neuropathy remains elusive, there's still hope. Here's why:

- Focus on What You Can Control: While the cause might be a mystery, the focus can shift to managing symptoms and improving your quality of life. This can involve lifestyle modifications, targeted supplements, and pain management strategies.

- Research on the Horizon: Scientists continue to delve deeper into the potential causes of idiopathic neuropathy. Advances in research might someday shed light on the underlying mechanisms and lead to more targeted treatments.

The RESTORE program acknowledges the challenges of navigating idiopathic neuropathy. We'll explore various strategies to support your nervous system health and empower you to become an active participant in your own wellness journey, even in the face of uncertainty.

If you have any of the risk factors for neuropathy, it's important to talk to your doctor about ways to reduce your risk of developing the condition. At Experience Health & Wellness Center, your source for chiropractic care and holistic wellness, we have personalized, holistic treatments available to help you manage the symptoms of neuropathy and improve your quality of life. In simpler terms, a holistic approach means treating the whole you, not just the symptoms. It considers how different aspects of your life – your diet, stress levels, sleep patterns – can all work together to influence your neuropathy and your overall health.

Defining Neuropathy

Neuropathy is a word that comes from two Greek words: neuro, meaning nerve, and pathy, meaning disease. Therefore, neuropathy literally means nerve disease.

However, neuropathy is not a single disease, but a group of conditions that have different causes and symptoms. Neuropathy can be classified into four categories, based on the type and location of the affected nerves:

- **Mononeuropathy** occurs when only one nerve is damaged, usually due to injury, compression, or infection. Carpal tunnel syndrome is a type of mononeuropathy that affects the median nerve in the wrist, causing numbness, tingling, and pain in the hand and fingers.
- **Polyneuropathy** is when many nerves are damaged, usually due to a systemic disease, such as diabetes, or exposure to toxins, such as alcohol or chemotherapy. Diabetic neuropathy is a type of polyneuropathy that affects the nerves in the feet and legs, causing loss of sensation, ulcers, and infections.

- **Autonomic neuropathy:** This is when the nerves that control the involuntary functions of the body, such as the heart, blood pressure, digestion, bladder, and sexual function, are damaged. For example, gastroparesis is a type of autonomic neuropathy that affects the nerves in the stomach, causing delayed emptying, nausea, vomiting, and bloating.
- **Cranial neuropathy:** This is when the nerves originating from the brain or the brainstem, such as the optic nerve, the facial nerve, or the auditory nerve, are damaged. For example, optic neuritis is a type of cranial neuropathy that affects the optic nerve, causing vision loss, pain, and inflammation.

Stories of Neuropathy Onset

Let's peek into the lives of everyday heroes, not superheroes, but ordinary folks like you and me, facing the unexpected challenge of peripheral neuropathy. These aren't just medical terms; they're real stories woven with hope, struggle, and, ultimately, the resilience of the human spirit.

Case 1: Barbara, the Dancing Queen - From Pirouettes to Pins and Needles

Barbara, a vibrant 62-year-old, had always prided herself on her active lifestyle. Zumba classes, weekend hikes, and spontaneous dance parties fueled her joy.

But then, a creeping numbness in her feet started stealing her rhythm. Walking became a chore, and the thought of dancing felt daunting. Fear and frustration painted her once-sunny disposition. It turned out to be diabetic neuropathy, a wake-up call that forced her to redefine "active."

Her journey involved embracing dietary changes, discovering gentle exercises, and finding new ways to express her zest for life. Today, Barbara may not pirouette like before, but she taps her feet with newfound appreciation, proving that joy comes in many forms.

Case 2: John, the Master Gardener - When Green Thumbs Turn Numb

John, a 58-year-old with a passion for nurturing life in his garden, felt a strange tingling in his fingertips while pruning roses. Soon, the vibrant colors of his flowers seemed muted, overshadowed by the growing numbness and weakness in his hands.

Gripping tools became difficult, and his cherished hobby felt like a burden. Diagnosed with carpal tunnel syndrome, a form of neuropathy, he feared losing his connection to the earth. But John wasn't one to give up.

He explored ergonomic tools, learned hand stretches, and even consulted a specialist for nerve-relieving techniques. Now, he cultivates not just his garden, but also his well-being, proving that adaptation can open doors to new possibilities.

Case 3: Maria, the Community Connector - From Coffee Klatsches to Coping with Clumsiness

Maria, a 70-year-old community organizer, known for her infectious laugh and warm gatherings, felt a change – a fumbling with coffee cups, a stumble on uneven ground. The diagnosis: peripheral neuropathy, attributed to her long-standing autoimmune condition. The fear of isolation loomed, threatening her cherished connections.

But Maria, ever resourceful, rallied. She sought support groups, explored mobility aids, and even organized "walking with canes" outings. Today, she navigates her world with grace and humor, proving that community spirit can blossom even in the face of challenges.

Remember, these are just glimpses into the diverse experiences of neuropathy. Each story holds a unique lesson, reminding us that hope and resilience can bloom even in the face of adversity.

The Costs of Ignoring Neuropathy

As you can see from these stories, neuropathy can have a significant impact on your life, affecting your physical, emotional, and social well-being. If you ignore your neuropathy, or delay seeking treatment, you may face serious consequences, such as:

- **Increased pain and discomfort.** Neuropathy can cause chronic and severe pain that can interfere with your daily activities and sleep quality. Some people describe the pain as burning, stabbing, shooting, or electric-like. The pain can also vary in intensity and frequency, making it hard to predict and manage.

Some people may also experience hypersensitivity, where even a light touch or temperature change can trigger pain. Neuropathy can also cause other unpleasant sensations, such as numbness, tingling, crawling, or itching, making you feel uncomfortable and restless.

- **Reduced function and mobility.**
  Neuropathy can impair your ability to
  perform simple tasks like walking, driving,
  typing, or holding objects. You may also lose
  your balance and coordination, increasing
  your risk of falls and injuries.

Neuropathy can also affect your organ functions, such
as digestion, bladder, heart, or sexual function. You
may experience symptoms such as constipation,
diarrhea, urinary incontinence, erectile dysfunction,
or irregular heartbeats. These symptoms can affect
your quality of life and your overall health.

- **Increased risk of complications and
  infections.** Neuropathy can make you more
  vulnerable to developing complications and
  infections, especially in your feet and legs.
  This is because neuropathy can reduce blood
  flow and impair wound healing.

You may also not notice any cuts, sores, or blisters on
your feet due to the loss of sensation. If left untreated,
these wounds can become infected, and in severe
cases, lead to gangrene or amputation. Neuropathy
can also increase your risk of developing other
conditions, such as Charcot foot, a deformity of the

foot bones and joints, ulcers, or open sores on the skin.

- **Reduced self-esteem and social interaction.** Neuropathy can affect your self-image and your confidence, making you feel embarrassed or ashamed of your condition. You may also feel isolated or depressed and avoid social activities or interactions.

Neuropathy can also affect your relationships, especially with your partner, if you have sexual dysfunction or intimacy issues. Neuropathy can also impact your work performance and limit your career opportunities or income.

As you can see, neuropathy can have severe and lasting consequences for your life if you ignore it or delay seeking treatment. That's why it's vital to take action as soon as possible and seek a comprehensive and effective solution for your neuropathy.

Early Detection Actions

One of the most important things you can do to prevent or relieve neuropathy is to detect it early. Early detection means identifying the signs and symptoms of neuropathy as soon as possible before they become severe or irreversible.

Early detection can help you avoid the costs and complications of ignoring neuropathy and give you a better chance of finding an effective treatment and improving your quality of life.

But how can you detect neuropathy early? Here are some tips and actions you can take:

Know your risk factors. Some people are more likely to develop neuropathy than others due to certain conditions or factors that can damage the nerves. These include diabetes, infections, injuries, toxins, medications, or genetic disorders.

If you have any of these risk factors, you should be more vigilant and aware of your nerve health. You should also try to control or reduce these risk factors by managing your blood sugar, treating your infections, avoiding injuries or toxins, reviewing your medications, or seeking genetic counseling.

Check your symptoms. Neuropathy can cause various symptoms, depending on the type and location of the affected nerves. Some common symptoms include numbness, tingling, pain, weakness, or loss of balance in your feet, legs, hands, or arms.

You may also have problems with your digestion, bladder, heart, or sexual function. If you notice these symptoms, you should not ignore them or dismiss them as normal or harmless. You should seek medical attention as soon as possible and get a proper diagnosis and evaluation of your nerve function.

Perform self-exams. One of the easiest and simplest ways to detect neuropathy early is to perform regular self-exams of your feet and legs, especially if you have diabetes or other risk factors. You should inspect your feet and legs every day, looking for any signs of injury, infection, or deformity, such as cuts, sores, blisters, swelling, redness, or changes in shape or color.

You should also test your sensation and reflexes by touching your feet with your fingers, a cotton ball, or a pin and checking if you can feel it. You should also check your temperature by comparing the warmth of your feet with the warmth of your hands or other parts of your body. If you find any abnormalities or differences, you should report them to a doctor immediately.

Use screening tools. Another way to detect neuropathy early is to use screening tools to measure your nerve function and identify abnormalities. These tools can include devices, tests, or questionnaires assessing your sensation, reflexes, strength, or pain.

For example, you can use a monofilament, a thin, flexible wire that can test your ability to feel pressure on your feet. You can also use a tuning fork, a metal instrument that can test your ability to feel vibration on your feet or legs. You can also use a questionnaire, such as the Michigan Neuropathy Screening Instrument, asking you questions about your symptoms, history, and risk factors.

You should use these tools regularly and follow the instructions carefully. If you get any abnormal or positive results, you should consult a chiropractor with extensive experience in treating neuropathy, like myself, for further evaluation and treatment.

These are some of the tips and actions you can take to detect neuropathy early and prevent or relieve its damage. By being proactive and aware of your nerve health, you can make a big difference in your life and enjoy a better quality of life.

The Painful Journey: How Neuropathy Affects Your Life

Neuropathy is not just a physical condition. It is also a painful journey that affects your life in many ways. In this section, I will share with you how neuropathy progresses, how it impacts different people, what are the emotional and physical costs of living with neuropathy, and what are some coping strategies that can help you manage your symptoms and improve your quality of life.

The Progression of Neuropathy

Neuropathy can progress at different rates and in different ways, depending on the cause and the type of nerve damage. Some people may experience symptoms gradually, while others may have a sudden onset.

Some people may have mild symptoms that do not interfere with their daily activities, while others may have severe symptoms that limit their function and mobility.

Others may have symptoms that come and go, while others may have constant and chronic symptoms. The progression of neuropathy can be influenced by several factors, such as:

- The underlying cause of the nerve damage and how well it is treated or controlled. For example, if neuropathy is caused by diabetes, keeping blood sugar levels within a healthy

range can slow down or prevent further nerve
damage.

- The type and location of the affected nerves
  and how much they are involved in the nerve
  damage. For example, if neuropathy affects
  the sensory nerves, it may cause more pain
  and numbness; if it affects the motor nerves,
  it may cause more weakness and muscle
  wasting.
- The individual's age, health status, and
  lifestyle. For example, older people, people
  with other medical conditions, and people
  who smoke or drink alcohol may have a
  faster or worse progression of neuropathy
  than younger, healthier, non-smoking, or
  non-drinking people.

The progression of neuropathy can be monitored by
regular check-ups with a doctor, who can perform
tests and exams to assess your nerve function and
identify any changes or complications.

At Experience, we conduct a comprehensive nerve
evaluation, which includes examining your
circulation and oxygenation levels. Here are some
other tests and exams we may perform:

- **Neurological exam:** This is a physical exam that evaluates your reflexes, muscle strength, sensation, balance, and coordination.
- **Blood tests:** These measure your blood sugar, vitamin levels, kidney function, liver function, and other indicators of your overall health and possible causes of neuropathy.
- **Nerve conduction studies:** These tests measure how fast and how well your nerves can transmit electrical signals. Electrodes are attached to your skin and deliver small shocks to stimulate your nerves. A machine records the response of your nerves and muscles.
- **Electromyography (EMG):** This test measures the electrical activity of your muscles. A thin needle is inserted into your muscle and records the signals your nerves send to your muscles when you contract them.
- **Imaging tests:** These tests use X-rays, ultrasound, CT scan, or MRI to create images of your nerves and other structures in your body. These can show any compression, inflammation, or injury to your nerves or the surrounding tissues.

By knowing how neuropathy progresses and how to monitor it, you can be more aware of your condition and seek appropriate treatment and care.

The Emotional and Physical Costs of Living with Neuropathy

Living with neuropathy can have a significant impact on your emotional and physical well-being. It can cause you to experience a range of negative emotions, such as:

- **Fear:** You may feel afraid of the unknown, of the future, of the complications, or the pain. You may worry about how neuropathy will affect your life, your work, your relationships, or your health. You may also fear that your condition will get worse or that you will lose your independence or dignity.
- **Anger:** You may feel angry at yourself, at others, or the world. You may blame yourself for causing or worsening your neuropathy or feel guilty for burdening your loved ones. You may also resent others for not understanding or supporting you or for having a better quality of life. You may also feel frustrated or helpless about your situation and lash out at those around you.

- **Sadness:** You may feel sad or depressed about your condition and how it has changed your life. You may grieve for the loss of your abilities, your function, your mobility, or your identity. You may also feel hopeless or worthless and lose interest or pleasure in the things you used to enjoy. You may also isolate yourself from others and withdraw from social activities or interactions.

- **Anxiety:** You may feel anxious or nervous about your condition and how it will affect you. You may have trouble sleeping, concentrating, or relaxing. You may also experience panic attacks, where you feel a sudden surge of fear accompanied by physical symptoms such as sweating, trembling, or palpitations. You may also develop phobias, such as fear of falling, fear of needles, or fear of crowds.

Neuropathy can also affect your physical health and cause you to experience various symptoms, such as:

- **Pain:** Neuropathy can cause chronic and severe pain that can interfere with your daily activities and sleep quality. Some people describe the pain as burning, stabbing, shooting, or electric-like. The pain can also vary in intensity and frequency, making it hard to predict and manage. Some people may also experience hypersensitivity, where even a light touch or temperature change can trigger pain.

- **Numbness**: Neuropathy can cause a loss of sensation or feeling in your affected areas, such as your feet, legs, hands, or arms. You may be unable to feel pain, heat, cold, or pressure. This can make you more prone to injuries, infections, or burns, as you may not notice any damage or discomfort. It can also affect your balance and coordination, as you may not be able to sense the position or movement of your limbs.

- **Weakness**: Neuropathy can cause a loss of strength or muscle mass in your affected areas, such as your feet, legs, hands, or arms. You may have trouble walking, standing, climbing stairs, or holding objects. You may also experience muscle cramps, spasms, or twitching. This can affect your mobility and function and increase your risk of falls and injuries.

- **Organ dysfunction:** Neuropathy can affect the nerves that control your involuntary functions, such as your digestion, bladder, heart, or sexual function. You may experience symptoms such as constipation, diarrhea, urinary incontinence, erectile dysfunction, or irregular heartbeats. These symptoms can affect your quality of life and your overall health.

Living with neuropathy can have serious and lasting consequences for your emotional and physical well-being. That's why seeking treatment and care as soon as possible and finding a comprehensive and effective solution for your neuropathy is vital.

Coping Strategies

Living with neuropathy can be challenging, but it doesn't have to be hopeless. There are some coping strategies that can help you manage your symptoms, improve your mood, and enhance your quality of life. Here are some tips and actions you can take:

- **Seek medical help:** The first and most crucial step is to seek medical help for your neuropathy. You should consult a professional as soon as you notice any signs or symptoms of neuropathy and get a proper diagnosis and evaluation of your nerve function.

You should also follow your holistic doctor's advice and take your prescribed supplements, therapy, or treatment. You should also monitor your condition and report any changes or complications to your doctor. Seeking medical help, especially from a holistic healthcare practitioner, can help prevent or relieve your pain and discomfort.

- **Seek emotional support:** Living with neuropathy can be emotionally draining, and you may need some support and encouragement from others. You should not be afraid or ashamed to ask for help or to share your feelings and experiences with someone you trust.

You can seek emotional support from your family, friends, or other people who care about you. You can also seek professional support from a counselor, therapist, or psychologist who can help you cope with your emotions and provide you with some tools and techniques to manage your stress and anxiety.

You can also seek peer support from other people who have neuropathy or who are going through similar challenges. You can join a support group online or in-person to connect with others, exchange information, advice, or stories, and feel less alone and isolated.

- **Seek lifestyle changes:** Living with neuropathy can also require some lifestyle changes that can help you improve your nerve health and function. You should adopt a healthy lifestyle that includes a balanced diet, regular exercise, and adequate sleep. You should also avoid or limit some unhealthy habits, such as smoking, drinking alcohol, or using drugs, that can worsen your nerve damage or interfere with your treatment.

You should also take care of your feet and legs, especially if you have diabetes or other risk factors. You should inspect your feet and legs every day, looking for any signs of injury, infection, or deformity, and treat them promptly. You should also wear comfortable shoes, socks, and gloves and protect your feet and legs from extreme temperatures or injuries. In addition, practice some relaxation techniques, such as meditation, yoga, or breathing exercises, that can help you calm your mind and body and reduce your pain and stress.

These are some of the coping strategies that can help you live with neuropathy and improve your quality of life. By following these tips and actions, you can make a positive difference in your life and enjoy a better quality of life.

Why Conventional Treatments Fail

If you have neuropathy, you may have tried some of the traditional approaches commonly prescribed or recommended by doctors or other health professionals. These approaches may include:

- **Medication:** This is the most common and widely used treatment for neuropathy. Medication can help relieve some of the symptoms of neuropathy, such as pain, inflammation, or depression. Some of the medications that are used for neuropathy include analgesics, anti-inflammatories, antidepressants, anticonvulsants, or opioids.
- **Surgery:** This is a more invasive and risky treatment for neuropathy. Surgery can help decompress or repair some of the damaged

nerves or remove some of the causes of nerve compression, such as tumors, cysts, or scar tissue. Some surgeries used for neuropathy include nerve release, nerve graft, or nerve transfer.

While these traditional approaches may have some benefits and advantages, they also have limitations and drawbacks, such as:

- **They are not effective for everyone.** Different people may respond differently to the same treatment, depending on their individual characteristics, such as their age, health status, genetics, or lifestyle. Some people may experience relief or improvement from a certain treatment, while others may not.
- **They are not specific for neuropathy.** Most of the traditional treatments for neuropathy are not designed or intended for neuropathy but for other conditions that may have similar symptoms, such as pain, inflammation, or depression. Therefore, they may not address the specific needs or challenges of neuropathy patients and may

not target the underlying causes of nerve damage.

- **They have side effects or complications.** Most of the traditional treatments for neuropathy have some potential side effects or complications that can affect the patient's health or quality of life. Some of the side effects or complications may include allergic reactions, addiction, dependency, tolerance, withdrawal, drowsiness, nausea, constipation, weight gain, liver damage, kidney damage, bleeding, infection, nerve damage, or scarring.

These are some of the limitations and drawbacks of the traditional approaches for neuropathy that can explain why they often fail to provide lasting and satisfactory results.

The Disappointment and Frustration of Conventional Treatments - Case Studies

While many seek solace in conventional medicine, some patients, like the individuals below, find themselves still yearning for a definitive answer:

Case 1: David, the Discouraged Diabetic - A Lingering Fire

David's diabetic neuropathy burns bright despite medication. The pills numb the pain, but the underlying cause – uncontrolled blood sugar – still simmers. He desperately searches for a way to extinguish the fire at its source, not just mask the flames.

Case 2: Margaret, the Wary Warrior - A Shadow of Improvement

Margaret's surgery provided a glimmer of hope, but the numbness returned, leaving her feeling like she's traded one monster for another. The lingering discomfort fuels her frustration, pushing her to explore alternative paths, determined to find a solution that truly conquers the beast.

Case 3: Michael, the Skeptical Seeker - A Tangled Web of Side Effects

Michael's medicine cabinet overflows, yet the side effects leave him feeling worse than the neuropathy itself. He's exhausted by the constant juggling act, yearning for a way to untangle the web of medications and find a solution that doesn't compromise his well-being.

These cases paint a stark reality – while conventional medicine offers valuable tools, some patients remain locked in a frustrating battle with neuropathy. Their stories echo a shared desire: a cure, a way to reclaim their lives from the clutches of this relentless condition.

It's crucial to remember that individual experiences vary greatly. While these portrayals highlight the limitations encountered by some, it's essential to acknowledge the successes achieved through conventional treatments for others. Consulting a healthcare professional for personalized guidance remains paramount.

The Dangers of Masking the Pain: Risks of Symptomatic Treatment

As you have seen in the previous section, conventional treatments for neuropathy often fail to provide lasting and satisfactory results. But there's another problem with these treatments that you need to be aware of. They are only symptomatic, meaning they only address the symptoms of neuropathy, not the root causes.

Symptomatic treatment can be useful in some situations, such as when you need to temporarily relieve your pain or discomfort or have no other option. However, relying on symptomatic treatment alone can be dangerous and can have severe consequences for your health and quality of life. Here are some of the risks of symptomatic treatment:

- **It can mask the underlying problem.** Symptomatic treatment can make you feel better, but it does not fix the problem that is causing your neuropathy. In fact, it can hide the problem and make you think that everything is fine when it's not. This can prevent you from seeking proper diagnosis and treatment and delay your recovery. It can also cause the problem to worsen and cause more damage to your nerves and other organs.

For example, if you have diabetic neuropathy and you take painkillers to ease your pain, you may not realize that your blood sugar is still high and that you need to control it better. This can lead to more nerve damage and increase your risk of developing other complications, such as kidney failure, blindness, or heart disease.

- **It can cause addiction or dependency.** Symptomatic treatment can be addictive, especially if you use opioids, such as morphine, oxycodone, or fentanyl, to relieve your pain. Opioids are powerful painkillers, but they also affect your brain and can make you feel euphoric, relaxed, or numb. This can make you want to use them more often or in higher doses to get the same effect.

Over time, you can develop a tolerance, meaning you need more opioids to feel the same relief. You can also develop a dependence, meaning you need opioids to function normally and avoid withdrawal symptoms, such as anxiety, nausea, or sweating.

Addiction and dependence can have serious consequences for your physical and mental health, such as liver damage, respiratory depression, overdose, depression, or suicide.

- **It can have side effects or interactions.** Symptomatic treatment can have side effects or interactions that can affect your health or quality of life. Some of the side effects or interactions may include allergic reactions, drowsiness, nausea, constipation, weight gain, liver damage, kidney damage, bleeding, infection, nerve damage, or scarring.

These side effects or interactions can be mild or severe and can vary from person to person, depending on your individual characteristics, such as your age, health status, genetics, or lifestyle. Some of the side effects or interactions can also interfere with your other medications, therapies, or treatments and reduce their effectiveness or safety.

For example, if you have chemotherapy-induced neuropathy and you take antidepressants to ease your pain, you may have trouble taking your chemotherapy drugs, as they may interact with your antidepressants and cause you to feel nauseous, anxious, or addicted.

These are some of the risks of symptomatic treatment that can explain why it's not enough and why you need to seek alternative solutions that address the root causes of neuropathy.

Beyond the Script: Exploring Cutting-Edge Solutions for Neuropathy

Living with the persistent pain, tingling, and numbness of neuropathy can feel like navigating a maze without a map. You've likely tried conventional medications or even surgery, but the relief might be fleeting, leaving you searching for more sustainable answers.

That's where exploring alternative avenues for healing comes in, offering a glimmer of hope on your journey toward reclaiming your well-being. Here are some natural, non-invasive, and non-addictive avenues we'll explore:

- **Chiropractic Care:** This holistic approach focuses on spinal alignment and nerve function. Gentle adjustments aim to improve nerve communication and reduce inflammation, potentially alleviating pain and promoting healing in some neuropathy cases. Imagine your spine as the highway for your nerves and chiropractic care as ensuring smooth information flow.
- **Physical Therapy:** Targeted exercises, modalities like electrical stimulation, and manual therapy techniques can improve circulation, reduce muscle tension, and promote nerve regeneration. Imagine gentle movements and specific exercises working their magic to enhance nerve function and mobility.
- **Targeted Supplements:** Specific vitamins, minerals, and herbal extracts have shown promise in supporting nerve health and reducing inflammation. These targeted

nutrients provide essential building blocks for your nervous system's repair and protection. However, consulting with a healthcare professional is crucial to ensure safe and appropriate supplementation based on your needs and medical history.

- **The Latest Non-invasive Technologies:** The field of neuropathy treatment is constantly evolving with emerging new technologies that offer promising options. These might include laser therapy, pulsed electromagnetic field therapy, or tissue regeneration technology like SoftWave therapy.

Remember, these are just a few examples. The key lies in individualization. We'll work together to identify the root cause of your neuropathy and tailor a RESTORE neuropathy program that resonates with your unique needs and preferences.

Navigating the Crossroads: When Neuropathy Demands Action

Imagine living your life with a constant companion – not a furry friend, but a persistent tingling, numbness, or pain that whispers, *"neuropathy."* You manage, you adjust, but lately, that whisper morphs into a shout. The pain intensifies, daily tasks become Herculean feats, and fear creeps in. This, my friend, is the crisis point.

Neuropathy doesn't have to become a life sentence, but ignoring its cries for help can lead to severe consequences. That's why understanding this crisis point is crucial. It's not just about pain escalation; it's about recognizing the potential domino effect on your well-being.

Here's what might signal the need for immediate action:

- **Worsening pain:** It's not just a dull ache anymore. The burning, stabbing, or shooting pain starts impacting your sleep, work, and overall quality of life.
- **Loss of balance and coordination:** Stumbling, falls, and clumsiness become more frequent, raising the risk of serious injuries.
- **Muscle weakness:** Simple tasks like buttoning a shirt or opening a jar feel like challenges, jeopardizing your independence.
- **Skin changes:** Numbness can mask injuries, leading to infections or ulcers that go unnoticed until it's too late.

- **Emotional toll:** Chronic pain, frustration, and fear can take a heavy toll on your mental and emotional well-being.

Now, this list isn't exhaustive. Every individual's journey with neuropathy is unique. But if you recognize these warning signs, don't wait for the crisis to peak. Seeking help and exploring treatment options, including those discussed in previous sections, can empower you to regain control and prevent further complications.

Ignoring the Ticking Clock: The Cost of Inaction in Neuropathy

Imagine a ticking clock, not on your wall, but inside you. Each tick represents the potential consequences of ignoring your neuropathy. While the present might feel manageable, the future can paint a different picture if left unaddressed.

We've talked about the crisis point, but the reality is the cost of inaction starts accumulating much earlier. It's not just about waiting for a major fall or a debilitating infection. Here's a glimpse into the hidden tolls of not taking action:

- **Physical decline:** Nerve damage progresses, potentially leading to muscle wasting, decreased mobility, and impaired balance, impacting your daily activities and independence.

- **Emotional burden:** Chronic pain, frustration, and anxiety take a toll on your mental well-being, affecting your quality of life and relationships.
- **Increased healthcare costs:** Untreated neuropathy can lead to complications requiring more intervention, potentially placing a strain on your finances and healthcare system.
- **Reduced productivity:** Difficulty concentrating, memory issues, and pain management can affect your work performance and earning potential.
- **Missed opportunities:** Fear and pain can restrict your ability to participate in activities you enjoy, limiting your life's experiences and fulfillment.

Remember, this isn't meant to scare you, but to empower you with information. Taking action doesn't mean waiting for the clock to strike midnight. Addressing your neuropathy early, through a personalized approach, like the RESTORE program, can help:

- Slow and potentially improve nerve damage.
- Manage pain effectively, improving your quality of life.
- Prevent complications and reduce healthcare costs.
- Maintain independence and return to the activities you love.
- Embrace a future filled with possibilities, not limitations.

By choosing to act, you're not just addressing a condition; you're investing in your well-being and reclaiming your life.

Remember, early intervention is key. Taking charge of your health today can make a significant difference in managing your neuropathy and preventing potential complications.

Freedom from Pain: Mary's Neuropathy Journey

"Before I came to Experience, I was suffering with severe neuropathy in my feet and lower legs. I couldn't walk, I couldn't cook, I couldn't clean my house, I couldn't do my laundry - I was miserable all the time with pain. It was difficult to sleep at night because my feet were numb and hurt constantly. I had been put on Gabapentin, which absolutely changed my whole personality. And I said no, I have to get off this. I'm not going to take medication. What can I do to naturally fix it? And I found Experience. Now I can walk, I can cook, I'm back into my exercise program, I can clean my house - I can do all the things I did before. My quality of life has improved 125%. It has been the blessing of my life to find the RESTORE program."

** Every patient's journey is unique. This testimonial does not guarantee similar results for others.*

ACTION STEP: Start a daily journal of your symptoms. This will allow you to more accurately sense your level of improvement when starting a neuropathy treatment regimen.

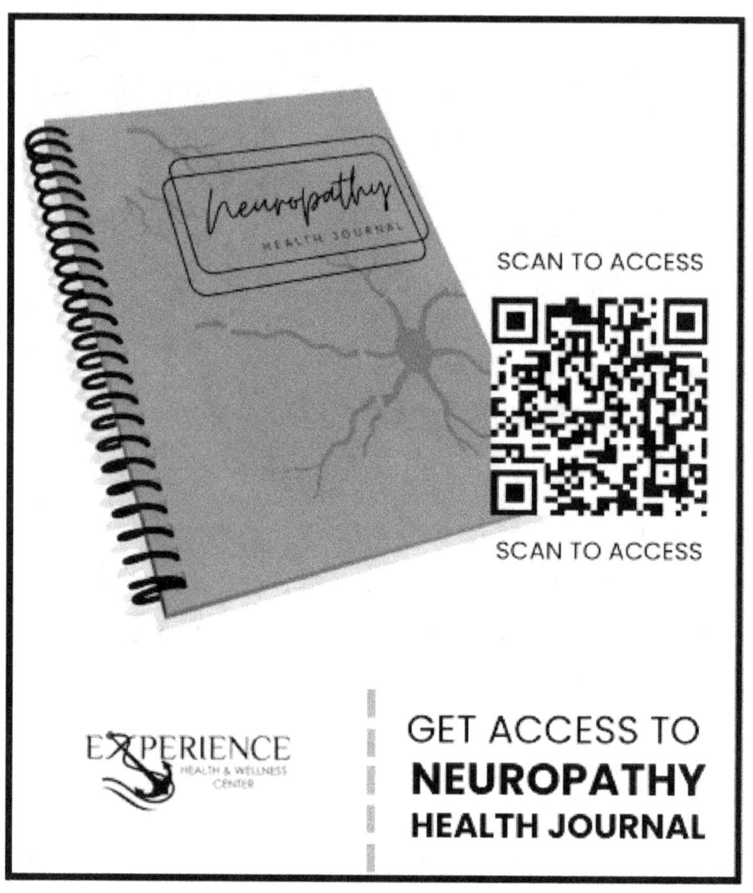

Unlock Your Path to Neuropathy Relief Now: Dial (239) 374-8654 to Speak With Us Today!

2

THE PROMISE OF R.E.S.T.O.R.E

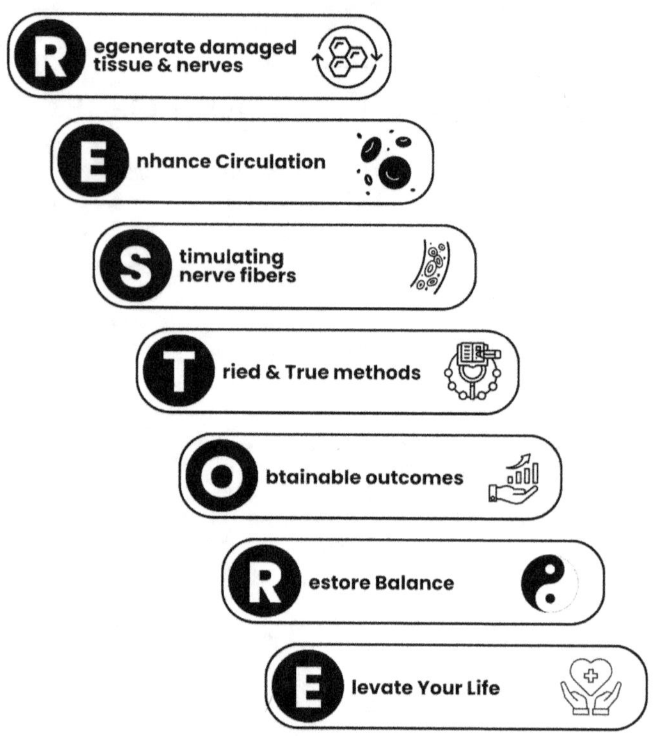

Peripheral neuropathy can feel like a relentless adversary, chipping away at your comfort and quality of life. Conventional treatments may offer only fleeting relief, leaving you feeling trapped in a constant cycle of medication and lingering discomfort. But here's the truth: there is hope.

The RESTORE Neuropathy Program is a beacon of possibility, crafted from years of experience and research. It's more than just a list of techniques – it's a powerful philosophy of healing targeting the underlying roots of neuropathy. I've strategically designed the name as a pathway to guide you forward:

- **R – Regenerate Damaged Tissue & Nerves:** Neuropathy isn't just about pain. It's about nerves that aren't firing correctly and tissues deprived of nourishment. Our program begins by fostering an environment where natural healing mechanisms can kick into gear.
- **E – Enhance Circulation:** For your nerves to function at their best, they need a steady flow of oxygen and nutrients. The methods we employ help open up pathways, giving your body a jumpstart in revitalizing damaged areas.
- **S – Stimulating Nerve Fibers:** Nerves that aren't properly used slowly lose their efficiency. It's the "use it or lose it" principle. We use targeted techniques to reignite these

slumbering nerves and encourage them to reconnect with your brain for clearer communication.

- **T – Tried & True Methods:** Don't mistake innovation for recklessness. Our program incorporates trusted approaches backed by both scientific research and years of helping patients navigate chronic neuropathy.

- **O – Obtainable Outcomes:** Results matter. I named this program RESTORE because that's the ultimate goal: restoring the vibrant life you deserve. This isn't about just living with neuropathy. It's about actively reversing its course.

- **R – Restore Balance:** Your nervous system interacts with every part of your body. Optimal nerve function helps everything operate harmoniously. RESTORE aims to rebuild a healthy foundation for wellness.

- **E – Elevate Your Life:** Our program isn't simply about physical improvements. It's about feeling confident in your body again, rediscovering activities you may have abandoned, and reconnecting with what truly sparks joy.

The RESTORE neuropathy program is not a miracle cure. It's a partnership between the team at Experience and you, where we share our deep understanding of neuropathy and proven treatment methods, while you commit to the steps that will reshape your journey toward better health.

Let's Talk About You

Remember those patient stories in Chapter 1? They could be your story. The tingling, the pain, the uncertainty... it doesn't have to be permanent. If this explanation of RESTORE has resonated even a little, it's worth the next step: let's discuss your path to healing.

Voices of Victory: When Neuropathy Takes a Backseat

Success stories aren't just about results – they're about transforming lives. These are voices of people just like you who've found a way out of the darkness of neuropathy. Let their courage and perseverance be your inspiration.

Michel: Reclaiming Life, One Step at a Time

"I can walk again. It's been absolutely amazing from where I came in to where I am now. I couldn't sit. I couldn't stand. I couldn't drive. I was out of work. I was in excruciating pain with several visits to and from the emergency room because of the pain. And within a month, I was back to being able to at least drive myself to my appointments and get back to work."

Michel's case reminds us how neuropathy's impacts go far beyond mere discomfort. When your movements are restricted, when pain dominates your days, fundamental needs and freedoms become jeopardized. Restoring the ability to enjoy daily routines and find independence makes every effort and challenge of healing utterly worthwhile.

Brittany: Embracing Hope and Healing

"From the moment I walked into Experience till the time I left, I was treated with love, respect and given high-quality care. The staff and the atmosphere of this place are so amazing and full of positive vibes and wonderful people. I would truly recommend anyone to this wonderful personally-owned business. It's the place to take your health to the next level."

Notice how Brittany emphasizes not just the treatment, but also the overall care she received. At its core, the RESTORE program isn't simply about medical interventions. It's about creating a welcoming, supportive environment where those fighting neuropathy can feel understood and empowered. We don't just care for your nerves. We care for the whole person.

Jack: Defying Expectations, Finding Improvement

"I remember sitting on the living room couch watching TV, feeling the toes in my right foot tingling. Then my left, and then slow but sure, they started to go numb. I saw a TV commercial for the EFC. It said it was holistic medicine. That caught my attention. So I made an appointment, and within the first month, I had feeling in my feet where I didn't have it before. Now my goal was to slow it down. Who would have guessed that I would've reversed it? So I'm pretty pleased with the whole deal. It's worth the effort. No two ways around it."

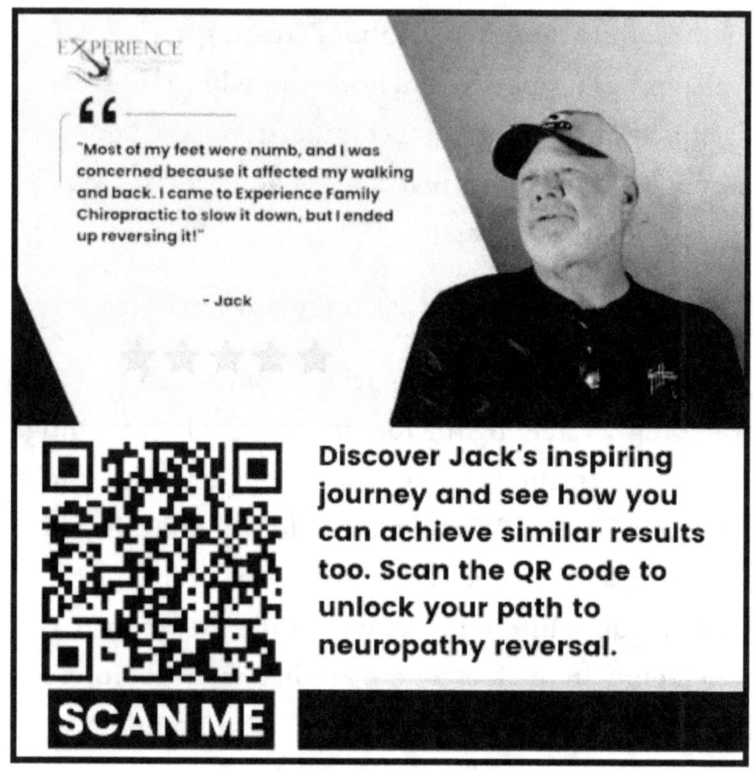

These testimonials reflect individual experiences and results, which may vary. They are not intended to represent or guarantee that everyone will achieve the same or similar outcomes.

Your Story Awaits

Michel, Brittany, and Jack represent just a piece of our community of patients taking back control from neuropathy. While everyone's path will be different, imagine these words reflecting your experience.

Imagine being the one who says, "I can walk again," "I'm back to doing what I love," and "I can finally feel optimism about the future."

The RESTORE neuropathy program stands ready to unlock that victory for you. Your journey toward healing takes courage, but you haven't come this far to stay stuck. Call us at (239) 374-8654 or visit our website, efchealth.com, to schedule a neuropathy evaluation, and let's write your success story together.

Please note that this evaluation is a starting point for understanding your individual needs and does not guarantee specific outcomes. Individual results may vary.

Benefits of a Holistic Approach to Neuropathy

Picture your body as a complex, interconnected network. Conventional medicine often excels at targeting isolated symptoms, like a mechanic attending to a single malfunctioning part. But with neuropathy, we need a different approach—one that sees the whole picture. This is what a holistic perspective offers.

When I use the term "holistic," I'm not just talking about incorporating lifestyle changes or alternative therapies. Holistic care delves into factors traditional treatments frequently overlook, including:

- **The Mind-Body Connection:** Chronic pain isn't solely physical. Mental and emotional well-being are inextricably linked to how we perceive discomfort. Your emotional state can worsen pain, and conversely, feeling stressed and anxious can aggravate existing neuropathy.

- **Hidden Culprits:** Neuropathy may have an obvious trigger, like diabetes or a medication side effect. But even then, other subtle imbalances could exacerbate the problem—things like nutritional deficiencies, gut health issues, or even unrecognized spinal misalignments impacting nerve signaling.

- **Individuality:** Nobody experiences neuropathy identically. Understanding what makes your case unique through detailed history and a thorough evaluation leads to tailored solutions, not just generic advice.

A tailored holistic approach offers the following advantages:

- **Root Cause Targeting:** We don't just mask symptoms; we strive to unwind the chain of events causing nerve damage or preventing healing. This leads to sustainable improvements, potentially offering relief not achieved through typical approaches.

- **Improved Overall Health:** When you address factors contributing to neuropathy, you may see surprising benefits ripple across your life. Patients often notice improved sleep, digestion, energy, and mental clarity, in addition to easing pain and numbness.

- **Empowerment and Autonomy:** Instead of feeling like a passive recipient of treatments, a holistic plan engages you in your own healing. Educating you about your condition and giving you tools fosters healthy decision-making for true well-being.

Promises of the RESTORE Neuropathy Program

At the heart of the RESTORE program is a multi-pronged strategy built on proven therapies customized to your specific challenges. While I can't guarantee any single outcome, here's what sets us apart and what patients typically strive towards:

- **Reduced Pain and Improved Function:** Our first aim is to bring you greater comfort and restore day-to-day abilities that may have been hampered. Techniques like chiropractic care, physical therapy, and emerging technologies all play a role in lessening your suffering.

- **Addressing Root Causes:** Through careful testing and examination, we pinpoint the underlying contributors to your neuropathy. Whether it's blood sugar optimization, nutritional restoration, or spinal adjustments, these customized interventions halt the disease process.

- **Healing Potential:** Your nerves weren't designed to stay damaged. The RESTORE Program seeks to ignite your body's regenerative abilities. Increased circulation, targeted tissue support, and the stimulation of nerves themselves facilitate your body's innate mending capabilities.

- **A Collaborative Approach:** Your participation is essential. This is not a "quick fix." We walk with you, provide guidance, track progress, and help you build habits that create lasting change. You gain both treatment AND the know-how to maintain the results long-term.

It's time to redefine what's possible in your life with neuropathy. Choose to move past just "coping" and embark on a path that offers the very real prospect of restoration.

More Than Management: Transformative Healing Starts Here

Picture this: neuropathy has chipped away at your life —affecting your mobility, your mood, and your sense of what's even possible. You've probably been tossed between treatment options that have provided some temporary relief, but never true and lasting change. It's easy to feel discouraged, trapped.

But what if there was a way to finally break this frustrating cycle?

That's the promise of transformative healing. It's about moving beyond mere symptom management and tapping into your body's own remarkable ability to mend itself. This isn't about false hope or miracles. This is about using the most proven scientific advancements, personalized for your unique needs.

A Roadmap for Your Own Transformation

Transformative healing doesn't come in a pill or a one-time treatment. It's a comprehensive approach, encompassing multiple areas:

- **Identifying the "Why":** This is detective work, looking at the factors driving your neuropathy—be it uncontrolled diabetes, spinal pressure on nerves, nutritional deficiencies, and sometimes even underlying conditions you didn't realize were connected.

- **Addressing the Damage:** Through innovative therapies, targeted exercises, and precise guidance, we aim to reduce inflammation, boost healthy circulation, and awaken nerve activity that's been compromised.

- **Building Sustainable Wellness:** From proper nutrition to techniques for stress management, we give you the tools and habits to prevent neuropathy from regaining a foothold. It's not just about feeling better now, but about making feeling better the new normal.

The most powerful resource in this journey isn't any technology or fancy equipment; it's you. Our program is designed to equip you with the knowledge and support needed to be active in your healing.

The path to this kind of freedom and well-being might be closer than you think. We want to understand your struggles, hear your story, and explore what transformative healing could look like for you.

If that sparks a glimmer of hope within you, call us at (239) 374-8654 or visit our website, efchealth.com, and schedule your neuropathy evaluation. This evaluation is designed to provide information and assess your individual needs. It's important to remember that individual results may vary, and this evaluation does not guarantee specific outcomes. This is your opportunity to discover what's possible and write your own success story.

From Bandaids to Breakthroughs: Moving Beyond Symptom Management

Too often, managing neuropathy means just numbing the pain—throwing a blanket over the fire instead of putting it out. Medications, creams, and even in some cases, injections, might momentarily mask discomfort, but they DON'T address the underlying reason your nerves are damaged or malfunctioning.

Think of it this way:

- **The Leaking Roof Analogy:** Imagine your roof keeps leaking, damaging your ceiling.

Patching up the wet spots provides temporary relief, but without fixing the actual hole in the roof, the problem returns. Neuropathy is similar. Pain medications are like those ceiling patches—they cover up a more significant issue but don't stop it.

- **The Weed That Won't Die:** You pull a weed out of your garden, but if the roots stay, it just grows back. With neuropathy, painkillers, injections, and topical treatments only tackle the above-ground "symptoms," not the root system responsible for your distress.

Root Causes: Where the Real Answers Lie

The secret to finding relief that lasts and potentially reversing damage lies in uncovering and addressing the root causes leading to your neuropathy. While these can vary greatly from person to person, here are some common root causes that need investigation:

- **Blood Sugar and Inflammation:** If you struggle with diabetes or even prediabetes, the excess sugar in your bloodstream isn't just taxing your organs; it's like tiny razor blades shredding your nerves. Uncontrolled inflammation throughout your body further exacerbates nerve damage.

- **Nutritional Gaps:** Your nerves, like all tissues, need specific nutrients to function and repair themselves. Vitamin B12 deficiencies are an often-overlooked contributor to poor nerve health, among other culprits. Addressing these gaps fuels your body's natural healing capabilities, reducing painful symptoms.

- **Spinal or Joint Misalignments:** The intricate network of nerves branches out from your spine. Even subtle pressure on spinal nerves or nerve irritation stemming from joint inflammation can throw off signals, leading to numbness, tingling, and weakness.

- **Lifestyle Factors:** Things like alcohol consumption, smoking, and lack of exercise can worsen neuropathy by reducing blood flow and further accelerating nerve damage. Taking an honest look at how lifestyle choices may be hindering your progress creates opportunities for impactful change.

Advantages of Root-Cause Healing

For many neuropathy sufferers, traditional approaches feel like an endless carousel of treatments with limited lasting success. It's tempting to lose hope.

But root-cause healing offers a fundamentally different pathway with distinct benefits:

1. **Lasting Relief, Not Just Temporary Fixes:** Remember our leaky roof analogy? With symptom-focused care, you're just patching up the damage again and again. But by addressing the source of the problem – the actual hole in the roof – you stop the cycle. This approach can halt further nerve damage and potentially improve past damage, unlocking sustainable relief.

2. **Improved Overall Health:** When you dive below the surface, you often find surprising ripple effects. For example, controlling blood sugar through diet and exercise may not only help your neuropathy but also reduce your risk of heart disease and boost your energy. Restoring proper spinal alignment and reducing inflammation might improve sleep and mental clarity alongside alleviating pain. Your "neuropathy treatment" becomes true wellness.

3. **Preventing Further Complications:** Untreated neuropathy isn't just about aches and numbness. Over time, it can leave you

prone to accidental cuts or burns, ulcers, infections, and in severe cases, even loss of feeling leading to injuries. Root-cause healing doesn't just treat what you feel right now—it reduces those risks down the road by improving nerve health and function.

4. **Reduced Medication Dependence:** While there may be situations where some symptom-relieving medication is temporarily needed, the goal of root cause treatment is to gradually reduce your reliance on these as your body heals. This means avoiding medication side effects, managing costs, and minimizing addictive potential, especially with opioids.

5. **True Empowerment:** The best treatments in the world don't work if you feel passive and uncertain. Understanding the "why" behind your neuropathy makes you an informed partner in your health journey. In the RESTORE program, we give you the tools to make lasting changes through the latest technology, diet, exercise, and lifestyle tweaks that keep your nerves working better even after your sessions are completed.

How to Embrace Root-Cause Healing: Your Invitation to Change

Maybe you recognize yourself in the stories we've shared. Perhaps you've seen fleeting glimmers of improvement with other treatments, but nothing that sticks. It's time to try a different road. Here's what embracing root-cause healing involves:

1. **Seek a Different Kind of Provider:** You deserve a healthcare provider who truly understands the complexities of neuropathy, who sees how many systems in your body can play a role, and who will take the time to listen to your specific challenges. You haven't failed—you just haven't yet found the right approach.

2. **Be Ready for Honest Investigation:** Uncovering root causes sometimes requires looking into parts of your health you may not have associated with neuropathy. Are you willing to explore food choices, previous injuries, stress levels, and perhaps even past therapies to fully understand what's causing your nerves to suffer? It's amazing what comes to light when you look with fresh, determined eyes.

3. **Prepare Yourself for Partnership:** True healing takes teamwork. Be prepared for honest conversations about your current habits, potential changes, and a new level of commitment. Expect education. Expect accountability. This isn't about magical shortcuts but about empowering you to work in tandem with your doctor to rewrite your story.

4. **Expect an Individualized Approach:** Nobody benefits from a generic plan. Be prepared for personalized care, whether that involves a blend of chiropractic adjustments, specific therapies, a customized nutrition plan, or all of the above. Root-cause healing is precision – finding what YOUR body needs.

5. **Don't Give Up on Hope:** You might feel skeptical, and some frustration is completely understandable. Healing from neuropathy rarely happens overnight. But when you target the source and not just the symptoms, lasting changes gradually evolve. Stay optimistic and consistent, celebrating even those small improvements as proof of your body's potential.

Taking the Next Step: Your Action Starts Here

We firmly believe that lasting neuropathy relief isn't found in just pills or fleeting interventions. It's about looking deeper, creating changes tailored to your body, and supporting your unique path back to health and mobility.

Let's discuss the nuances of your case, delve into potential problem areas, and discuss root-cause solutions through the lens of your individual needs. While we are committed to helping you achieve your best possible outcome, it's important to understand that individual results may vary. Our approach is tailored to each patient's unique needs, but we cannot guarantee specific results. Call us today at (239) 374-8654 or sign up for our free masterclass to learn more about your neuropathy and how we can help. You deserve to get your life back. Let's make it happen!

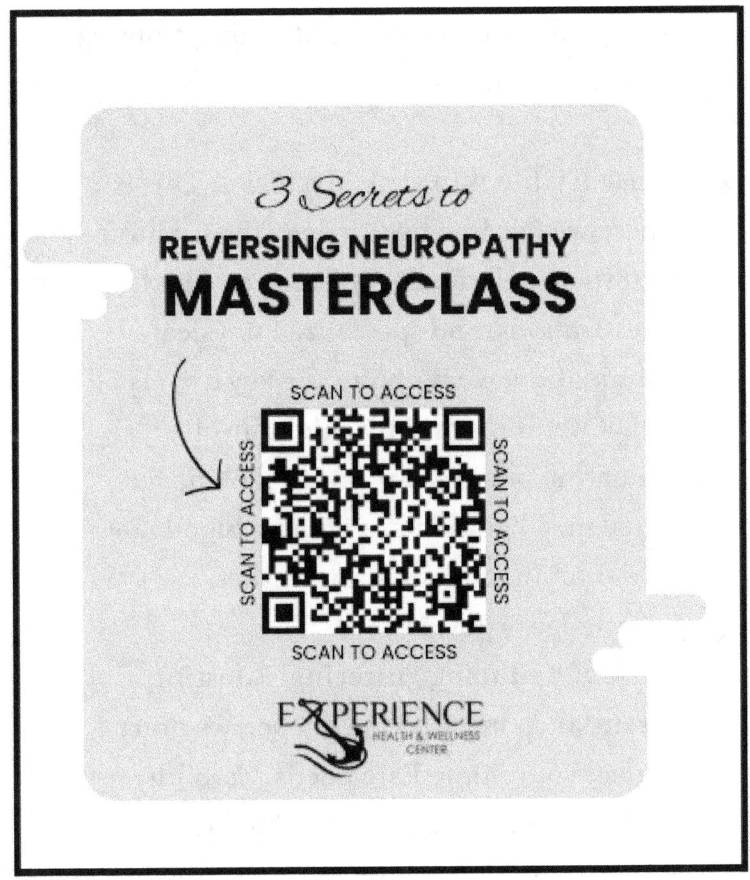

Your Roadmap to Recovery: The Path of the RESTORE Neuropathy Program

For too long, neuropathy might have felt like navigating a confusing maze with dead ends at every turn. The RESTORE program offers a structured, multi-faceted roadmap to lead you towards not just coping, but truly finding relief and restoring your well-being. Imagine this path unfolding in phases, each with its own focus:

- **Phase 1: Unlocking the Mysteries:** This is where we become health detectives. Through your thorough medical history, targeted investigations, and specialized physical examination, we pinpoint the key drivers of YOUR neuropathy. This might involve evaluating blood sugar levels, looking for spinal misalignments, assessing blood flow, or identifying inflammatory issues. Knowledge is power.
- **Phase 2: Reducing Suffering, Boosting Potential:** While digging deeper, we don't neglect your immediate needs. Carefully chosen therapies, physical or lifestyle adjustments, or even temporary supplements can all play a role in providing much-needed comfort while targeting the root of your problem. You might experience less tingling, a resurgence of energy, or simply the easing of daily pain—laying the foundation for deeper healing.
- **Phase 3: Reviving Nerves, Igniting Health:** Think of your nerves as resilient but delicate

wires that have been frayed. Here, we use tailored therapies, advanced technology, and personalized exercises designed to restore nerve function and boost blood flow to create a healing environment. As your nerves reawaken and repair, your body reclaims its natural health.

- **Phase 4: Sustainability and Freedom:** Our goal is to move you beyond merely feeling good when you come in for an appointment —it's about empowering you to maintain and continue improving on your own. This phase encompasses the tools and practices to keep your neuropathy in check long-term, through diet, movement, stress management, and the newfound understanding of what keeps your body thriving.

Beyond Symptom Relief: The Rewards of Complete Healing

Choosing this path means looking forward to more than just a dulling of pain. As your nerves revitalize, as inflammation subsides, and as your body functions closer to its optimum, imagine a life full of these possibilities:

- **Rediscovering Mobility and Activity:** Walking without stumbling, enjoying sports or hobbies that bring you joy, feeling confident in your balance...these become possible goals when your nerves start sending reliable signals to your muscles and brain.

- **Sleep That Actually Restores:** Imagine waking up feeling refreshed, not with aching legs or buzzing feet robbing you of rest. Reduced pain and optimized nerve function unlock a night of true recuperation and daytime energy.

- **Less Medication, More Control:** Over time, your reliance on painkillers and other medications is significantly reduced or even eliminated, minimizing costs, side effects, and your sense of reliance on temporary fixes.

- **A Brighter Outlook:** As your body repairs, your spirit naturally follows. With less physical burden and renewed freedom, a brighter outlook, renewed passion, and greater mental clarity often find their way back into your daily experience.

Keep in mind: every recovery is unique, but when you embrace holistic support and root-cause healing, these results are the prize awaiting on the other side of your struggle.

Preparing for the Journey: Setting Realistic Expectations

Your RESTORE neuropathy program is tailored to you, as is your timeline for improvement. But here's what to expect about the process itself:

- **Honesty and Partnership:** Be truthful about your past experiences, what you've tried, and your expectations. In return, we will be transparent about your plan, likely steps, and potential challenges. We only succeed when we're a true team.
- **Consistency is Key:** This isn't a one-shot deal. Think of it as training your body to reclaim its natural capabilities. Consistent adherence to your personalized plan, dietary changes, and at-home exercise or support are vital to long-term success.
- **Patience Amidst Progress:** Nerve healing takes time. Setbacks may occur when addressing stubborn or chronic cases.

However, when you stick with it, celebrate those "baby steps" of improvement, and trust that this approach allows for more profound change than you may have experienced before.

Choosing the RESTORE method is about becoming empowered. It's recognizing that your well-being stems from the choices you make, not just the care you receive.

From Numbness to Normalcy: Joni's Neuropathy Journey

"Dr. Clark's neuropathy program is amazing. I've regained control over my life. The tingling and numbness in my feet are gone, and I can finally enjoy walking, exercising, and playing with my grandchildren again. It's truly been life-changing."

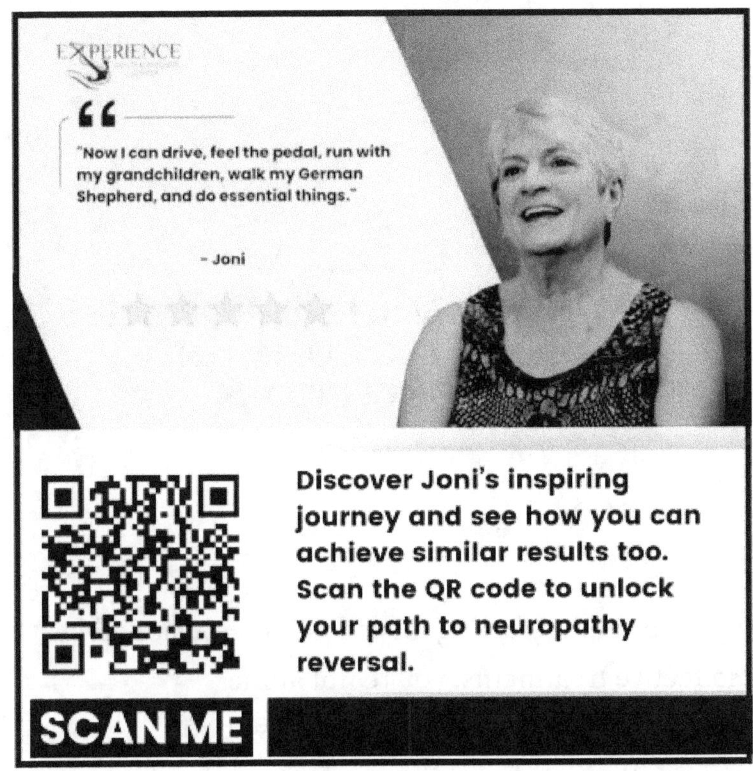

** Individual results may vary.*

Unlock Your Path to Neuropathy Relief Now: Dial (239) 374-8654 to Speak With Us Today!

3

THE TRUTH ABOUT NEUROPATHY: DISPELLING COMMON MISCONCEPTIONS

If you're tired of feeling misled and disillusioned by ineffective treatments, you're not alone. Unfortunately, many popular beliefs about neuropathy simply aren't true. This section exposes common myths and offers a reality check based on sound science and experience.

Myth #1: "Neuropathy is just a normal part of aging."

The Reality: While it's true that neuropathy becomes more common with age, it's absolutely NOT a natural consequence of getting older. Often, other health conditions like diabetes, circulation issues, or lifestyle factors are responsible for the nerve damage associated with aging.

Why This Myth Matters: Dismissing neuropathy as a "senior problem" creates an attitude of acceptance instead of a search for solutions. Believing it's unavoidable deters people from seeking help, allowing underlying causes to continue and worsen over time.

Myth #2: "If I have neuropathy, I'm destined for a wheelchair or amputation."

The Reality: While these are severe potential outcomes, they are NOT the default prognosis for everyone with neuropathy. Many different nerves are affected in various ways. Early intervention, addressing root causes, and making positive lifestyle changes can significantly slow the progression of neuropathy. Some individuals even experience noticeable improvement in their symptoms and nerve function.

Why This Myth Matters: Fear is a powerful motivator, but one that often drives towards hasty or incorrect decisions. If someone operates from this kind of anxiety, they might opt for invasive procedures too quickly or be susceptible to false promises when they feel desperate.

Myth #3: "Medications are the only way to manage neuropathy."

The Reality: While medication can be vital in alleviating certain symptoms, it rarely addresses the core cause of nerve dysfunction. When medications mask the problem, not solve it, they come with long-term risks and limitations. Holistic, root-cause approaches aim to create a situation where medication may be decreased or unnecessary altogether.

Why This Myth Matters: Putting all of your faith in a pill promotes a passive attitude towards neuropathy. Medications have their place, but informed patients realize there's more to genuine healing than relying solely on pharmaceutical remedies.

Myth #4: "You can 'detox' your way out of neuropathy."

The Reality: "Detoxes" promoting special diets, juices, or cleanses might sound appealing, but they often capitalize on false claims and fear-mongering. While healthy eating supports overall well-being, there's no scientific evidence these can miraculously reverse nerve damage.

Why This Myth Matters: Quick fixes are tempting, but rarely yield real results. These fads exploit the desperation people feel, promising an end to pain without any true effort on the patient's part. Instead of wasting time and money on unproven "cures," seek out therapies with demonstrated effectiveness.

Myth #5: "Once nerves are damaged, there's nothing you can do.

The Reality: Your nervous system has the potential for impressive regeneration. While this can take time and commitment, your body often holds surprising healing abilities. With the right approaches targeting blood flow, inflammation, and direct nerve stimulation, you can encourage this process, not hinder it.

Why This Myth Matters: It creates a bleak mindset that sabotages any effort to improve. True progress begins with believing it's even possible. Embracing your body's healing potential paves the way toward making the necessary changes and committing to treatment.

This is just a glimpse into the misinformation circulating about neuropathy. Be wary of any treatment promising instant, effortless fixes or preying on fear with overstated worst-case scenarios. Having worked with countless neuropathy patients, I'm here to share the knowledge I've gained, debunking those common myths that often hinder true healing.

Voices of Change: When Stories Shatter Neuropathy Myths

We've busted the myths, but sometimes, understanding what's NOT true still doesn't illuminate what IS. These real-life stories showcase the potential held within individuals struggling with neuropathy. It's not about magic tricks; it's about tapping into what your body can accomplish with the right support.

Turning Back the Clock – Barbara's Fight Against 'Normal' Deterioration

Barbara, at 62, thought the increasing numbness in her feet was the beginning of the end. "Getting old stinks," she'd sigh to her friends. But something didn't sit right. After getting properly diagnosed with early diabetic neuropathy, she overhauled her diet, incorporated exercises specifically for circulation, and was thrilled to see a gradual but clear improvement! Her energy increased, and she reconnected with her love of long walks with her grandkids.

Stepping Away from Fear – Jake Defies Limitations

When Jake's pain was so severe that even driving short distances was impossible, a sense of panic about being housebound overwhelmed him. An acquaintance even warned him it'd be the wheelchair next. However, through an individualized treatment plan that combined chiropractic care, specialized therapies, and addressing overlooked nutritional deficiencies, he gained strength and mobility. While Jake will always manage certain aspects of his neuropathy, that fear? Completely erased!

Empty Promises, Empty Wallet – Sarah Learns the Hard Way

Sarah stumbled upon a social media ad promising a miracle neuropathy cleanse, claiming fast and painless results. Out of desperation, she splurged on the overpriced supplements and followed the restrictive diet...only to see zero change. Feeling even more disheartened, her search for real answers nearly stalled until she reached out for a true consultation about root causes.

Awakening Healing – Miguel Discovers Renewed Hope

After several disappointing medical consultations, Miguel nearly settled for a lifetime of painkillers and a slow decline in his active lifestyle. Then, he discovered an approach that looked beyond symptom management. Through consistent treatment focused on boosting nerve function and tailored support, he gained remarkable strength in his legs and his spirit. "It's a marathon, not a sprint," he always says, but one he now tackles with optimism.

Remember, your story doesn't have to follow a path dictated by myths and misinformation. Be inspired by these individual victories and challenge your own beliefs about what's possible. You deserve the chance to find the solutions that unlock a better quality of life, free from the constraints of neuropathy.

Beyond Frustration: Why Misinformation About Neuropathy Is Dangerous

When your quality of life is on the line, navigating the healthcare world can be daunting. With neuropathy, it's worse. You likely hear conflicting advice, encounter vague promises that turn out empty, or fall prey to scare tactics used to market questionable "cures."

But this isn't just annoying; it's genuinely harmful. Here's why misinformation should be seen as more than just a source of frustration:

- **Delays Real Help:** The longer you chase down ineffective strategies, the more precious time slips away. While you exhaust yourself testing unproven supplements or temporary Band-Aid solutions, the underlying causes of your neuropathy are allowed to worsen. This makes future treatment harder and decreases the likelihood of significant improvement.

- **Fuels Desperation:** Feeling like you're running out of options can make you vulnerable to anyone touting a seemingly quick fix. Even the most discerning person can make decisions driven by desperation when in enough pain or fear. This often leads to financial loss on expensive but pointless products and procedures with lasting negative mental and emotional consequences.

- **Undermines Trust:** Every time you experience disappointment due to a treatment based on misinformation, your trust in legitimate healthcare professionals erodes. This fuels skepticism about even appropriate or potentially beneficial treatments and ultimately, hurts your well-being.

- **Can Have Physical Repercussions:**
  Remember, neuropathy isn't just about
  unpleasant sensations. It reflects a
  malfunction in your nervous system, putting
  you at higher risk for injuries and infections.
  Ignoring these red flags while focusing solely
  on a temporary reduction in pain through
  deceptive remedies can create long-term
  damage.

- **Hinders Empowerment:** Accurate
  information makes you an active partner in
  your health. If you base your decisions on
  misconceptions, you lose agency.
  Understanding your neuropathy empowers
  you to seek effective care, advocate for
  yourself, and regain control over those areas
  you can affect.

Protecting yourself from this deluge of
misinformation isn't always easy. It requires a critical
mindset and commitment to asking the right
questions. Fortunately, you have allies. Partnering
with us at Experience, who treats you as an individual
with unique concerns – can ensure you have science-
backed guidance at all stages of your journey.

Building Immunity to Misinformation: Your Toolkit

Think of yourself as a savvy healthcare detective. Don't blindly accept every headline or persuasive advertisement. Let's equip you with the tools to distinguish between sound facts and false promises.

Questions to Ask Yourself

- Does it sound too good to be true? Grand claims of instantaneous results, "secret cures" your regular doctor isn't aware of, or guarantees of relief for even the most complex cases should all be red flags.
- Where's the evidence? Reputable treatment providers cite reliable clinical research or case studies that back up their methods. Vague testimonials or references to "ancient wisdom" without specific supporting details should not inspire confidence.
- Who's the seller? A reputable healthcare professional is transparent about their credentials, practice setting, and focuses on treating you holistically, not just selling you a specific product or device.
- What's the fine print? Any credible offer for treatments comes with both potential

benefits and limitations explained clearly. Be wary of anything claiming only positive effects without any honest discussions of what it does NOT address.

Beyond Your Gut Feelings

- Discuss with your doctor. Before starting a new supplement, trying a trendy technique, or pursuing out-of-pocket services, run it by a trusted doctor familiar with your case. They can give you science-based feedback to protect your health and wallet.
- Research reputable sources. Organizations like the American Diabetes Association (if relevant to your case) or trustworthy websites like the Mayo Clinic are good starting points. Here's a few more:
  - MedlinePlus
  - Department of Health and Human Services (HHS)
  - Centers for Disease Control and Prevention (CDC)
  - American Medical Association (AMA)
  - National Institutes of Health (NIH)

Remember, focus on material that addresses complex causes of neuropathy, not simplified fixes.

- Be wary of social media hype. Platforms often prioritize what's engaging and shareable, NOT what's factually sound. Question dramatic before/after stories and seek professional opinions to get the full picture.

The Power of Informed Partnership

The most valuable defense against misinformation is a trusting relationship with a healthcare provider dedicated to both cutting-edge care and open communication. Look for these hallmarks in your care:

- **No Shame or Judgement:** It's okay (and normal!) to have tried things based on what you saw or were told. A good doctor respects your journey and focuses on empowering you to better understand what's beneficial or harmful moving forward.
- **Individualized Assessment:** Generic or cookie-cutter solutions rarely lead to long-term improvements. Your treatment plan should feel crafted uniquely for YOU, not something pulled off a pamphlet.

- **Ongoing Education:** You deserve to know why treatments are suggested, their potential limitations, and what progress looks like. Feeling like you're part of a team builds trust and allows you to confidently filter outside information through what you've learned from your own experience.

We believe you deserve reliable and compassionate care. Stay vigilant, ask questions, and lean on credible sources when looking for solutions. This fight against misinformation is essential in your path to true neuropathy relief.

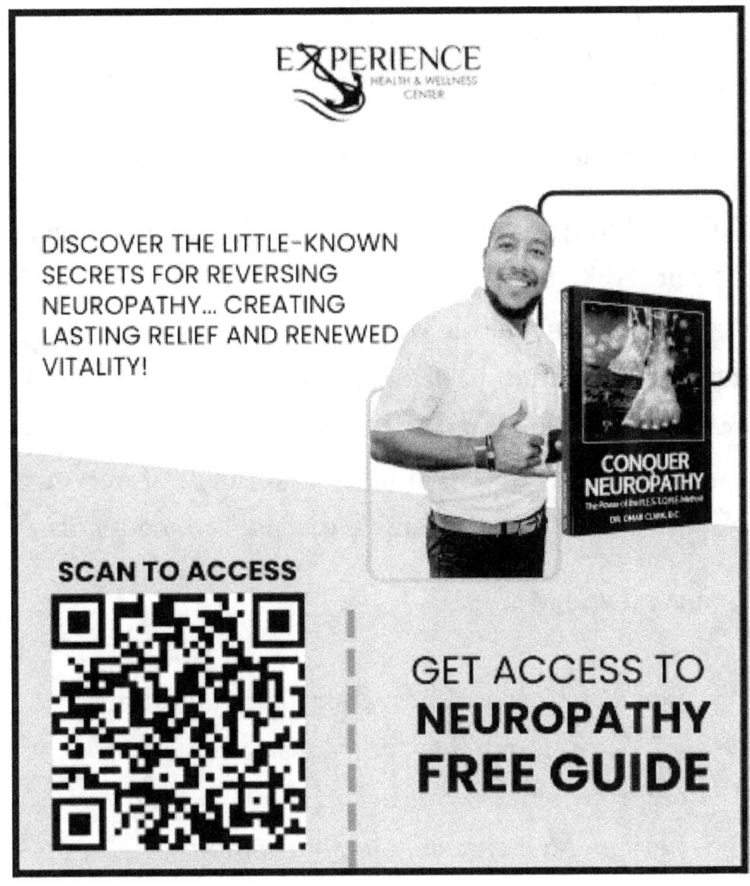

Untangling the Misconceptions About Neuropathy

For anyone with neuropathy, it's not just the symptoms that are tough; it's often the lack of clear understanding. Friends, family, and even some medical professionals downplay its complexity or perpetuate inaccuracies about what it means to have this challenging condition. Dispelling those myths starts here.

Misconception #1: "Neuropathy is a single disease."

Think of neuropathy like the engine light on your car dashboard. It signals a problem, but that light alone doesn't tell a mechanic what to fix. Similarly, nerve dysfunction comes in diverse forms, requiring careful evaluation to understand the specific "why" behind it. This involves understanding a bit about your nervous system. Here's why the "single disease" concept fails:

1. Nerve Type Matters:

- Sensory Nerves: These deliver signals about what you touch, feel, and sense about your environment to your brain. Damaged sensory nerves cause that classic neuropathy numbness or tingling, as well as loss of balance and sensitivity to temperature.
- Motor Nerves: These control your muscles, allowing for movement. When these malfunction, weakness, cramping, and difficulty with fine motor skills can occur.
- Autonomic Nerves: This branch unconsciously regulates vital functions like digestion, heart rate, blood pressure, and even sexual response. Dysfunctional

autonomic nerves cause seemingly disconnected yet problematic symptoms.

2. Root Causes Diverge: What can damage or dysregulate these various nerves? Here's a PARTIAL list, each influencing treatment radically:

- Metabolic: Uncontrolled conditions like diabetes and pre-diabetes create toxic blood chemistry that assaults nerves.
- Toxicity: Metal exposure, medication side effects, or overconsumption of alcohol all harm nerves in unique ways.
- Physical: Nerve compression from spinal stenosis or injuries can impact motor nerves primarily. This often coexists with metabolic-driven neuropathy.
- Nutritional: A diet lacking essentials like B vitamins or an inability to absorb these efficiently leaves nerves vulnerable.
- Autoimmune: When your immune system goes rogue, it can attack specific nerves, leading to unusual manifestations beyond the common sensations.

3. The Symptom Trap: "Numbness & Tingling" only captures sensory nerve issues. Symptoms of autonomic or motor dysfunction are mistakenly dismissed as unrelated problems. This traps patients in endless cycles of seeking specialist appointments while nobody connects the dots to their broader nervous system health.

Consequences of the "Single Disease" View

- Diagnostic Frustration: If it's not immediately obvious (like severe uncontrolled diabetes), finding the right root cause takes time and often, specialized assessment beyond standard testing.
- Wasted Treatments: A pain-focused approach or generic therapy that worked for a friend's diabetic neuropathy is useless for someone whose issue stems from pinched nerves in their spine.
- Exhausted Spirits: As solutions fail, patients often assume nothing works for them when perhaps, nothing APPROPRIATE has even been tried yet.

Accurate classification through thorough assessment gives you a powerful advantage - it's the starting line for targeted care that moves beyond just covering up a flashing dashboard warning light, and actually focuses on what repairs are needed.

Misconception #2: "Only diabetics and the elderly get neuropathy."

While it's true that both the elderly and those with diabetes are statistically at higher risk, these classifications only tell a sliver of the story. Let's look at what science and clinical experience reveal:

1. The Hidden Drivers of Risk:

- Beyond High Blood Sugar: Pre-diabetes, insulin resistance, or impaired glucose tolerance aren't as dramatic as uncontrolled blood sugar, yet still create progressive nerve damage. Undiagnosed or dismissed as "inevitable" due to family history, this silently sets the stage for neuropathy even in seemingly otherwise healthy individuals.
- Overlooking Common Medications: Medications used for everything from depression to high blood pressure and even certain antibiotic classes can have neurotoxic side effects. Many are considered generally safe, but individual susceptibility or existing underlying health issues create risk.
- Age Isn't Just About Wear and Tear: Yes, nerves naturally change with the passage of time. However, lifestyle factors accelerate this

deterioration. Decades of poor diet, inactivity, and chronic stress create the perfect internal environment for nerves to falter. This contributes to why younger and younger individuals develop neuropathy.

- Hidden Toxin Burden: The world is sadly more polluted than ever. Heavy metals through diet, occupational exposure, or even seemingly benign sources like dental fillings can accumulate silently. Nerves are exceptionally sensitive to even low-level chronic toxin load.

2. The Overlooked Mimics:

- Lyme Disease: Left untreated, this insidious bacterial infection can create devastating neurological issues mimicking other illnesses. Joint pain, muscle weakness, and neuropathy-like symptoms often lead to misdiagnosis and delays in accurate treatment.
- Vitamin Deficiencies Beyond B12: While lack of B12 causes well-documented nerve issues, insufficiency in essential nutrients like B6, Folate, Vitamin D, and others can cause neurological changes ranging from subtle to

profound. This is especially common after bariatric surgery.

- Untreated Trauma and Spinal Issues: Even old injuries, disc problems, or chronic postural habits can pinch or restrict blood flow to nerves. Treating underlying root causes like low vitamins are useless without addressing these structural factors.
- Autoimmunity: When your body attacks itself, nerves aren't exempt. A growing number of conditions like Hashimoto's thyroiditis, systemic lupus, and vasculitis can be responsible for confusing symptoms mistakenly deemed as 'neuropathy.'

Consequences of the "Only Diabetic and Elderly" Assumption

- Unnecessary Suffering: Young adults are told it's impossible they have "real neuropathy" as doctors disregard root causes unique to their generation.
- Delaying Essential Care: Symptoms progress when the underlying driver is ignored. Lyme is the perfect example where prompt treatment is key.

- Missed Connection to Other Disorders: If your neuropathy has an autoimmune cause, managing THAT becomes a top priority to halt nerve damage.

The good news: A more inclusive view of neuropathy opens doors to discovering answers and reversing dysfunction even in atypical cases. It requires both knowledge and looking beyond conventional boxes.

Misconception #3: "It's all about the numbness and tingling."

Imagine an iceberg. The visible portion represents only a fraction of the true threat lurking beneath the waves. Similarly, classic neuropathy symptoms are surface-level clues that much deeper harm could be happening within your nervous system. Why this matters:

1. Neuropathy Attacks More Than Just Sensory Nerves:

- Motor Nerve Damage: This isn't always a dramatic loss of movement. Instead, look for: Unexplained muscle weakness, cramps, or foot drop. Difficulty buttoning up shirts, loss of grip strength, and even frequent tripping over unseen obstacles can all stem from weakened nerve signaling to muscles.

- Autonomic Nerves: This invisible branch often creates the most bizarre symptoms: sudden spikes in heart rate, random blood pressure changes, bowel or bladder incontinence, difficulty sweating or adjusting to temperatures – all are possible neurological issues disguised as something else.

2. Symptom Severity Doesn't Equal True Problem:

Sometimes, burning pain in the feet is the loudest complaint and may indeed be severe. But what if, under the surface, silent damage to nerves controlling digestion or immune function is happening concurrently? It's impossible to prioritize treatments while missing the full picture.

3. "Weird" Symptoms Get Dismissed:

Unexplained rashes, sexual dysfunction, sensitivity to certain textures, a sudden inability to tolerate a familiar food - these aren't merely oddities. Each can be a clue pointing to nerve dysfunction in ways most individuals and even doctors won't connect readily.

Consequences of Focusing on the Obvious

- Misdiagnosis Trap: Each new symptom gets a separate evaluation. A cardiologist looks at the heart, a gastroenterologist focuses on the gut... yet an underlying neurological issue continues to fester unaddressed.
- Treatment Misfire: When the origin is mistaken, therapies only mask, not fix. Acid reflux pills won't correct autonomic nerve damage causing digestive issues.
- Lost Time: The body has incredible reserves and often compensates when nerves misfire. However, these compensations become increasingly unsustainable. This could mean sudden falls, unexplained organ problems, or a dramatic acceleration in pain severity later on.

This is why at Experience, we take a broad, personalized approach to assessing potential neuropathy cases. Your symptom list matters, but it serves as a map pointing us toward deeper investigation through advanced testing and examination, not a self-contained diagnosis.

Misconception #4: "If your blood tests are normal, you don't have neuropathy."

Picture standard medical bloodwork as a basic roadworthiness check on your car. It flags obvious issues – a blown tire, empty oil tank, a dead battery. These demand immediate attention, just as high blood sugar or severe anemia necessitate prompt care. However, your nervous system functions more like a finely tuned computer network than a combustion engine. Subtle malfunctions aren't readily observed with these rudimentary tests.

1. Bloodwork Has Its Limits:

- Focus on Pathology: Standard bloodwork is a screening tool. It detects if you're outside the range indicating possible disease (high cholesterol, blood cell defects, etc.). But 'normal' doesn't mean 'optimal' when it comes to nerve function, nor does it uncover gradual declines. Early, reversible nerve changes occur long before a reading raises alarms.
- Static Snapshot: Tests capture a moment in time. Issues related to nutrient absorption, immune function, or fluctuations driven by diet aren't reflected accurately. Inflammation is another key driver of neuropathy; many basic blood tests miss these crucial markers.

2. Specialized Neuropathy Assessment: This goes beyond simple 'checks':

- Nerve Conduction Studies: These directly measure how fast, robustly, and accurately electrical signals travel along your nerves. A skilled practitioner interprets not just if results are 'abnormal,' but identifies patterns pointing towards the type of nerve damage involved (sensory vs. motor, large vs. small fiber).

- Advanced Metabolic Markers: Beyond basic glucose, advanced panels look at how well you utilize blood sugar, your insulin response, and inflammation within blood vessels. A nuanced picture of potential early metabolic nerve damage emerges.

- Nutrient Levels: A standard panel shows if you're severely deficient. Assessing how well your body absorbs vitamins, your genetic propensity for poor utilization, and how levels reflect within tissues (not just in the blood) reveals subtle clues often overlooked.

3. False Reassurance vs. Proactive Detection:

The goal isn't simply diagnosis, but to uncover the root causes to treat BEFORE irreversible damage happens. Waiting until advanced neuropathy appears on standard bloodwork could lead to:

- Dismissed Suffering: Burning feet in a healthy 40-year-old woman is brushed off, when perhaps specialized testing would illuminate pre-diabetic metabolic shifts or B12 absorption issues reversible in early stages.
- Delay in Lifesaving Care: Unstable blood sugar spikes and low-grade inflammation could silently erode nerves for years before reaching 'abnormal' thresholds.
- Missing Treatment Opportunities: If an autoimmune cause exists, the earlier it's detected, the more aggressive intervention has a better chance of mitigating long-term nerve destruction.

The right tests can translate vague complaints into targeted answers. It's about empowering you to navigate a path built on early intervention, not crisis management.

Misconception #5: "Treatment is only about controlling symptoms, not getting better."

Think of a forest fire. Medications for neuropathy work like tossing buckets of water at the visible flames – it brings temporary relief, but the underlying problem still smolders. However, a multi-pronged approach combines those necessary tactics with addressing the factors that allowed the fire to take hold in the first place. This creates the foundation for sustainable change. Here's a closer look:

1. Your Nerves Are Built to Repair:

Unlike tissues permanently damaged by trauma, nerves hold amazing regenerative capacity. But, they need the right conditions to rebuild themselves. Focusing only on masking pain doesn't support them in this complex healing process. It's akin to taking painkillers after a broken bone while ignoring that it needs to be set and casted.

2. Root Cause: The Key to True Improvement:

- Uncontrolled Diabetes: Yes, strict blood sugar regulation can reverse painful changes over time. But what about optimizing nutrient absorption, which is often poor in such patients, or tackling insulin resistance? This creates faster and more enduring effects.
- Inflammation: This is like gasoline on the neuropathy fire. Diet, specific

supplementation, and uncovering sources of hidden inflammation create a less damaging environment your nerves can heal within.

- Targeted Nutrients: Deficiencies, and even insufficiencies within "normal" ranges, can starve nerves of what they need. Replacing these fuels their regenerative processes.

3. Therapies Beyond Symptoms:

Innovative technologies stimulate dormant nerves, boost cell activity, and increase circulation to revitalize tissues. Alongside proper physical and chiropractic care, this isn't about merely feeling better, but creating measurable changes in how those nerves function.

Consequences of the "Only Symptom Control" Belief

- Temporary Relief: The moment medication stops, or life stress flares up, pain comes roaring back. This reinforces that patients are helpless victims of their bodies.
- Progressive Worsening: While symptoms wax and wane, the underlying disease (if present) and nerve destruction proceed unhindered.
- Missed Out Possibilities: There's a huge difference between reduced numbness and

restored feeling back in an affected area, even partially. This translates to less risk of injury, and the return of simple pleasures like feeling the ground beneath your feet.

Healing IS possible. The body has remarkable power when fueled and supported appropriately. Don't settle for a life defined by chronic pain and fear of what comes next. This is the cornerstone of the RESTORE method - moving you beyond just management towards the possibility of genuinely reclaiming your well-being.

Instant Relief vs. Sustainable Healing

If you've stumbled down the rabbit hole of internet "cures" or been tempted by infomercials promising effortless relief, you know the frustration of dashed hopes. Sadly, these quick fixes exploit desperation and lack critical understanding of what lasting changes entails.

When dealing with a chronic condition like neuropathy, "feeling better" almost instantly should spark suspicion, not relief. Why? Here's a breakdown of why those fast changes tend to be illusions:

Symptom Masking

Let's expose an unfortunate truth about many products marketed as a quick answer to neuropathy pain – they're the equivalent of putting a fancy bandaid on a deep wound. Here's a closer look at why the symptom-masking approach will backfire in the long run:

1. The Pain Deception:

- How Painkillers Work: Most OTC drugs (Ibuprofen, etc.) target inflammation pathways. When inflammation underlies nerve irritation, this can provide temporary relief. More powerful prescription meds block your brain's ability to interpret the pain signal itself. While sometimes necessary in situations of extreme pain, this is akin to cutting the wires to a smoke alarm instead of putting out the fire.
- Masking vs. Treating: If all discomfort vanishes instantly, you falsely assume that the product is curing you. Instead, while you no longer feel it, nerve damage may actually increase unnoticed due to continuing root causes (e.g., unmanaged blood sugar spikes) or neglecting crucial lifestyle changes.

2. Short-Term Gains, Long-Term Problems:

- Side Effects: Even OTC meds put a strain on your liver and kidneys over time. Gut health disruptions common with these drugs worsen nutrient absorption, which fuels your nerves. Masking discomfort with pills can prevent you from making positive diet shifts.

- Tolerance: Your body gets used to many meds. Soon, your dose stops working as well, creating an escalating cycle where you crave stronger ones while still making zero progress on healing. The higher the medication dose, the bigger the risk profile becomes.

- Missed Out Healing: While numbing allows brief moments of activity, true progress depends on identifying why the malfunction and inflammation happen in the first place. That often requires some level of discomfort to drive investigating root causes instead of popping a pill!

3. Over-the-Counter Doesn't Always Equal Safe:

- Herbals & "Naturals": While marketed as gentle, unregulated supplements/creams sometimes contain potent unlisted ingredients with risks if mixed with other medications or conditions. Always inform your doctor of EVERYTHING you take, not just prescriptions.

- Interactions: Often, those desperately seeking solutions try multiple quick fixes at once. Certain OTC drugs mixed with specific supplements can be dangerous or worsen side effects. Without transparent guidance, it's an uncontrolled experiment on your health!

IMPORTANT: I'm not advocating ditching ALL symptom relief. Sometimes, temporary use is necessary during difficult pain or treatment initiation. However, these tools must be part of a larger strategy focused on treating the source of your distress, not just covering it up.

Temporary Blood Flow Improvements

Let's explore why focusing on short-lived blood flow improvements is a losing battle when treating neuropathy. Think of it this way:

Imagine a drought-stricken plant – its leaves are wilting, and it's clearly suffering. Just adding a trickle of water makes a tiny, temporary difference. Yes, there's momentary relief, but without addressing the lack of consistent water (and perhaps nutrients and soil issues), the plant won't truly recover.

Same goes with neuropathy. Nerves become starved when blood flow is inadequate, hindering the delivery of oxygen and nutrients, and removal of metabolic waste.

Here's the breakdown:

1. Vasodilation Isn't Enough:

- Brief Surge: "Vasodilatory" essentially means that substances cause a quick burst of blood vessel widening. Certain herbs, caffeine, and even hot compresses do this temporarily. This may feel good as more blood rushes in, but it doesn't solve the underlying problems causing compromised circulation in the first place.
- Deeper Causes: Persistent blood vessel constriction comes from chronic inflammation, oxidative stress (unregulated "rust" damaging cells), and metabolic disruption like that which happens in poor glycemic control. It is impossible to sustainably overcome these without root-cause intervention.

2. Band-Aid Solutions:

- Fleeting Improvement: You may feel less numb when blood flow surges momentarily during your cream application. But a few hours later, the effect vanishes, and your body is back where it started – with underlying, smoldering dysfunction.
- False Hope: These slight changes trick you into thinking you've stumbled upon something amazing. It fosters a dependence on continuous re-application and delays in seeking comprehensive solutions focused on restoring sustainable healthy circulation.

3. Blood Vessels in Neuropathy Aren't Just Narrowed:

- Endothelial Damage: The lining of blood vessels (especially tiny ones serving nerves) becomes inflamed and stiff in metabolic disease and as toxic burden accrues. It isn't just about squeezing a tight pipe, but a pipe itself that functions improperly.
- Blood Viscosity: The actual thickness and composition of your blood matters. Issues like poor hydration, excess inflammatory fats

in your diet, and even nutrient deficiencies make blood stickier, hampering flow no matter how "wide" the vessel tries to be.

Addressing circulation concerns in neuropathy requires:

- **Blood Sugar Regulation:** If underlying, this must be prioritized through consistent diet and appropriate support/monitoring.
- **Reducing Inflammation:** Targeted nutrition, specific botanicals, and uncovering trigger foods all play a part in creating a healthier environment for your blood vessels.
- **Targeted Therapies:** Innovative technologies go beyond "feeling warm." Properly used, they stimulate vascular regrowth, repair damaged linings, and promote improved oxygen delivery at the tissue level.

The right plan considers ALL contributing factors to poor circulation, not a temporary boost masking the problem.

Untreated Root Cause

While instant relief is thrilling, if your blood sugar remains volatile, nutrient deficiencies persist, or that pinched spinal nerve doesn't get relieved, your neuropathy WILL eventually worsen regardless of fleeting moments of calm.

Here's how to understand this crucial fact:

1. The Fire Inside: Imagine a small campfire within your body. It might represent chronic uncontrolled blood sugar (like in pre-diabetes), a lurking immune flare due to ongoing gut problems, or an insidious hidden source of inflammation caused by past injury.

- Symptom Relief is Dowsing the Flames: If you throw water on those flames, you get instant, dramatic relief. Perhaps a pain medication masks how it feels (equivalent to water for short-lived comfort). It doesn't fix what ignited or fuels the fire.
- Embers Smolder Underneath: While you are basking in that moment of comfort, the smoldering fire beneath stays active. Its damage now goes undetected. Over time, that fire can unexpectedly surge again, or leave a trail of increasing destruction (worsened neuropathy) even when masked fairly well.

2. Examples of Root Causes Quick Fixes Don't Impact:

- Metabolic Chaos: If pre-diabetic or poorly managed insulin resistance lies at the heart of your nerve damage, temporary relief tricks you into thinking the diet changes/exercise you need to prioritize are optional. You may even gain weight due to false security while the real disease escalates.
- Autoimmune Neuropathy: If an attack on your nerves (due to Hashimoto's thyroid disease, Vasculitis, etc.) is missed, even fantastic symptom control leads to devastating progression unless that autoimmune condition is identified and actively treated.
- Structural Dysfunction: A pinched nerve in your spine from chronic postural problems or undetected past injury cannot be fixed by pills or creams. Temporary numbing lets you overexert (due to feeling less pain), actively fueling the nerve irritation and setting you up for long-term worsened issues.

3. Consequences of Ignoring Root Causes:

- Misinformed Decisions: Feeling great despite no actual improvements influences whether you keep doctor's appointments, consider further testing, or stick to lifestyle changes (that would really help but feel less critical since you seem better).
- Progressive Injury: While you feel okay, nerves silently wither. It leads to sudden falls when muscle weakness finally hits a tipping point, unrecognized infections from lost sensation, and neuropathic pain that becomes intractable when only treated late-stage.
- Missing Treatment Window: For some root causes, the sooner targeted action is taken, the greater the possibility of full or even partial nerve function restoration. If you get complacent in a cycle of fleeting fixes, this opportunity becomes heartbreakingly lost.

Actual progress begins with identifying the "WHY" behind your neuropathy, not fleeting bursts of feeling better that disguise ongoing deterioration.

Stories of Failed Quick Fixes

Here are snapshots of real journeys to illustrate why

those who abandon the search for overnight results gain far more in the long run:

- Sarah's Miracle Supplement Trap: For months, Sarah spent hundreds of dollars on pills praised in internet hype groups. Temporary improvements always disappeared, leaving her deflated and with less money for things shown to support recovery, including targeted supplements or consistent physical therapy.
- Tom's Device Frenzy: Desperate to avoid medication, Tom tried every electric stimulation gadget out there. Short bursts of relief were exciting, but unsustainable. It left him broke and no closer to figuring out WHY his neuropathy started in the first place.
- Michelle's Breakthrough Moment: After failed "miracle" diets and cleanses, Michelle hesitated when a new chiropractor offered a plan spanning weeks. The right blend of therapies, blood sugar management, and nutritional corrections gave her the most noticeable and LASTING change she'd ever experienced.

Remember, quick fixes thrive on impulsive decisions driven by false promises. Don't be discouraged by these setbacks. It's not your fault for hoping for an easier route. Shifting your mindset and investing in evidence-based treatments is where the potential for truly getting better resides.

Shifting Beyond Fleeting Fixes – The Sustainable Healing Mindset

We've exposed the pitfalls of chasing elusive cures. If these missteps fill you with disappointment, there's an empowering truth on the other side: Your well-being isn't about one grand moment of reversal, but rather, consistent choices built on informed action that leads to genuine healing.

Here's what adopting this attitude entails:

- **Understanding the 'Marathon' Nature:** Healing damaged nerves, reversing root-cause imbalances, and rebuilding function takes more than days or weeks, especially in long-standing cases. It's like training for a marathon, not a sprint – focus on progress, not instant results.
- **Commitment to the Process:** You become an active participant, not a passive recipient.

This may mean dietary shifts, targeted physical therapy, learning stress-reducing techniques,... It's not about quick-fix ease, but consistent action tailored to your needs.

- **Prioritizing Root-Cause Treatment:** Alongside targeted care to soothe existing symptoms, we'll focus on uncovering and addressing the WHY behind your nerve dysfunction. This is what ensures your improvement continues even after treatments are completed.

Realistic Expectations – The Promise of True Progress

Sustainable recovery looks different for everyone, depending on the root cause and how far the damage has progressed. Realistic goals provide motivation, not discouragement.

- **Improved Everyday Function:** This might mean walking with less risk of falls, regaining finger dexterity to open jars without struggles, or sleeping more soundly due to lessened night pain. We focus on what matters most in your life.
- **Gradual Strength Restoration:** It's a journey, not an overnight switch. You may be

surprised how small tweaks in gait or movement lead to major stability leaps as nerves are supported and revitalized over time.

- **Increased Well-Being Beyond the Pain:** Reducing dependence on meds, optimizing blood sugar, or uncovering hidden contributors (like vitamin deficiencies) doesn't just benefit your neuropathy. Your overall health, energy, and mental clarity often receive a welcome boost.

Your Ally In This Journey

This path can be challenging but immensely rewarding. I'm not here to promise miracles, but to be your knowledgeable, supportive guide. It means:

- **Honest Evaluation:** Understanding your history and utilizing accurate tests is crucial for creating an individualized care plan. No generic approach or misleading hype here.
- **Evidence-Based Care:** I draw from up-to-date research, proven technologies, and clinical experience to craft your plan. This builds trust in knowing it's based on sound science, not fleeting fads.

- **Openness to Adjustments:** Healing isn't linear. The right care plan adapts alongside your progress and individual responses. Your feedback matters as we collaborate towards your improvement.

Are you ready to ditch the cycle of short-lived hope, and embrace the journey towards the truly lasting solutions your body is capable of? Call us today at (239) 374-8654 or visit our website efchealth.com/neuropathy.

When "Nerves Meet Lifestyle" – The Impact You Can Control

Often, people are told their neuropathy is solely about their age, their condition (like diabetes), or simply bad luck. While those play a role, there's an overlooked piece you have direct control over - your lifestyle. It's not about blame, but empowerment through understanding HOW this matters.

Lifestyle: The Amplifier of Neuropathy

Think of this as a volume knob: Even if predisposed to neuropathy, having a healthy lifestyle keeps the volume low – symptoms might be mild or completely absent. But harmful daily habits turn that volume up, significantly escalating nerve damage and impacting how treatable your condition ultimately is.

Here's why your choices truly matter:

- **Blood Sugar Balance:** Even within "normal" blood test ranges, what you eat creates subtle spikes and dips influencing nerve health. Poor insulin sensitivity is like rocket fuel for neuropathy, even if diabetes isn't on your chart yet.
- **Inflammation's Impact:** Diet, stress, gut health, etc., generate constant low-grade inflammation in the body. This directly worsens neuropathic pain, erodes your blood vessel integrity, and sabotages healing at the cellular level.
- **Nerves Need Nourishment:** Vitamin deficiencies (especially B Vitamins), toxic overload, and poor nutrient absorption create environments where nerves simply cannot function properly, no matter what other treatments you implement.

Real-World Examples: See Why Lifestyle Matters

Understanding goes deeper with seeing this connection in action:

- The Office Worker on a Soda Habit: Chronically high consumption elevates blood sugar long after that initial spike, even outside those diagnosed with diabetes. Couple this with a sedentary job, and your nerve health recipe is primed for trouble.
- The Stressed-Out 'Healthy Eater': A seemingly nutritious plant-based diet won't help if underlying gut dysfunction isn't addressed. Poor nutrient absorption can cause significant deficiencies even when eating well. Chronic stress worsens neuropathy independently.
- The Retired Couch Potato: Lack of movement creates blood flow stagnation, poor muscle support around nerves (contributing to compression), and a steady erosion of balance and nerve-muscle feedback. The more inactive, the faster that worsening happens.

Important Note: Lifestyle as a component of treatment doesn't mean perfection. It means strategic, gradual shifts based on what is realistic for YOU. The focus is on progress, not guilt. We work together to assess your starting point and find leverage points that are the most likely to produce results and be sustainable.

The Ripple Effect: The Benefits of Lifestyle Adjustments

Lifestyle changes shouldn't feel like punishment; they're tools of self-care that directly improve the function of your nervous system. While individual recommendations will always be personalized, let's understand their power when incorporated into your program. Imagine experiencing:

- **Increased Stability & Endurance:** Diet changes that stabilize blood sugar, targeted movement plans, and addressing any nutritional deficiencies all build muscle support and increase safety through better mobility and fewer energy crashes.
- **Improved Sleep & Mental Clarity:** When pain wanes naturally and blood sugar fluctuations reduce, quality sleep returns. Often, brain fog lifts, improving mood and memory in subtle yet noticeable ways alongside direct treatment.

- **Reduced Dependence on Medication:** This becomes achievable alongside consistent progress. Over time, with reduced nerve irritation and inflammation, reliance on both prescription and OTC drugs will be possible even if complete cessation isn't your goal.
- **Renewed Hope & Self-Efficacy:** Taking ownership through informed action fosters a sense of agency. It becomes the antithesis of the helplessness or "just dealing with it" attitude that neuropathy often wrongly brings.

Practical Recommendations: Small Changes, Big Impact

Don't feel overwhelmed. Positive transformation stems from tailored guidance and focusing on what will impact YOUR symptoms the fastest. Here are common adjustments for many neuropathy patients:

- **Dietary Shifts:** No one-size-fits-all. This ranges from blood sugar balance plans to inflammation-reducing options, addressing food sensitivities to promote improved absorption of critical nutrients.
- **Targeted Supplements:** Often, addressing deficiencies or using natural compounds

proven to enhance nerve function jumpstarts healing. This complements other therapies, allowing them to work even better for YOUR body.

- **Mindset Mastery:** Stress significantly worsens neuropathy and perception of pain. Techniques to manage daily stress aren't just 'feel good' add-ons. Think of it as strengthening your inner shield against negative triggers.

- **Customized Movement Therapy:** Exercise is powerful, but the wrong kind can make you worse. We carefully identify movements to safely restore flexibility, strength, and stimulate repair of nerves and blood vessels.

It's about more than just following directions and checking off boxes. With guidance, you understand WHY specific changes lead to improved well-being. We work together to tailor these recommendations so they work for your life, building confidence and long-term sustainability for managing your neuropathy.

Experience Health: Where My Neuropathy Disappeared

"I went hoping for whatever help they could provide for my neuropathy. I was in constant pain with severe numbness and was using a cane because my balance was also off. I wasn't sure their RESTORE program would work, but I took the plunge and was determined to follow the program they had laid out for me. I even took everything with me on vacation. IT WORKED! My persistence paid off! They were supportive, friendly, and professional. It took a year, but my neuropathy is almost totally gone! If you have neuropathy, check out Experience Health. The doctors and their staff are great!" - Mary B.

Results are not typical. Your experience may vary.

ACTION STEP: Take our free Nerve Damage Evaluation by scanning this code:

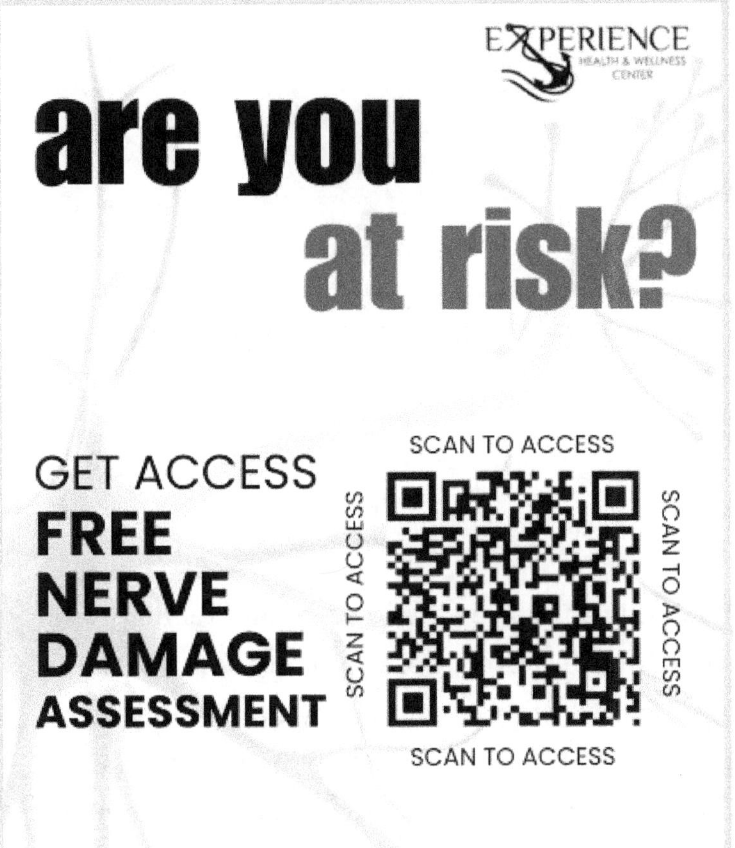

Unlock Your Path to Neuropathy Relief Now: Dial (239) 374-8654 to Speak With Us Today!

4

———

BLOOD SUGAR CHAOS: YOUR NERVES IN THE CROSSHAIRS

We live in a world awash in sugar and refined carbohydrates. Even those vigilant about eating "healthy" are often unknowingly overloading their bodies with hidden culprits fueling blood sugar imbalance. Sadly, this constant metabolic tug of war doesn't just lead to extra pounds or an energy crash after indulging in a treat. Unstable blood sugar paves a direct path to nerve damage and peripheral neuropathy.

Think of your nervous system like a complex electrical network. Those circuits can't fire correctly or stay healthy when exposed to constant "voltage surges" in the form of blood sugar crashes and highs. Imagine if you constantly plugged and unplugged your electronics or flooded the system with too much power... you'd expect damage! This chapter will illuminate this insidious process and the steps you can take to safeguard your nerve health.

Preview: The "Why" Behind the Chaos

We'll dissect the following to truly understand the threat uncontrolled blood sugar poses to your nerves:

- **The Typical American Diet's Fault:** This isn't just about donuts! Our environment and food choices, even supposedly "low-fat" ones, create constant pressure on our body's ability to keep blood sugar steady. Here are some common culprits to watch out for:
- **Sugary drinks:** Soda, sports drinks, and fruit juices are loaded with added sugars.
- **Refined carbohydrates:** White bread, pasta, pastries, and white rice are quickly digested, causing blood sugar spikes.
- **Processed meats:** Hot dogs, deli meats, and bacon are often high in sodium and unhealthy fats.
- **Fried foods:** French fries, onion rings, and fried snacks are loaded with unhealthy fats and can contribute to inflammation.
- **Packaged snacks:** Cookies, chips, and crackers are often high in refined

carbohydrates, unhealthy fats, and added sodium.

- **Insulin - Friend or Foe?:** This hormone is meant to be your guardian, but overwork and abuse turn it from protector to threat. How this happens is critical to understand for prevention.
- **Beyond Diabetes:** Even if you don't have a blood sugar diagnosis, early damage and neuropathy occur silently at levels considered "fine" through routine testing. Learn the crucial warning signs.

Understanding this issue opens the door to preventative action. It's about far more than avoiding desserts – it's about empowering you to make targeted choices that foster true stability and safeguard your well-being.

Dissecting the Standard American Diet: Why "Normal" Isn't Healthy

What most consider everyday food choices actually creates an environment of metabolic unrest in your body. This isn't simply about willpower or calorie counting. Let's explore how even with the best intentions, common patterns can lead to blood sugar imbalances that silently pave the way for the development of neuropathy.

A. Deceptive "Health" Foods:

"Low Fat" Doesn't Equal Blood Sugar Friendly: Decades of focus on fat reduction led to added sugar and refined carbs to improve taste. That low-fat cookie may have fewer calories than the full-fat version, but it leads to a more severe blood sugar spike and crash.

"Whole Wheat" Isn't Always What It Seems: Modern wheat is processed for fluffy textures, losing much of its fiber benefit. This means fast digestion turning straight into blood sugar, regardless of it being labeled "whole wheat" bread.

Hidden Sugars Everywhere: Sauces, dressings, even "savory" items sneak in sugar under various names. Constant small doses, even if you don't eat much dessert, add up, forcing your body to relentlessly work to keep blood sugar in check.

B. It's Not Just About Sweets:

Portion Distortion: Even with healthy food, the concept of "supersized" meals creates a blood sugar surge. This overwhelms even a healthy person's ability to process everything efficiently, especially if the meal lacks proper balance of protein and healthy fats to slow digestion.

Carbohydrate Overload: While essential nutrients, our bodies didn't evolve to handle the constant intake of refined grains, even whole ones. Many people simply lack the enzyme capacity for large amounts of bread, pasta, and even seemingly healthy sweet potatoes.

The Snacking Trap: Instead of defined meals, constant grazing is disastrous. Even "healthy" nuts or fruit cause repeated insulin release, never giving your body a rest or allowing it to tap into its energy reserves.

Important Note: This isn't about blaming individuals. Our food industry is designed to promote overconsumption and addiction. But, understanding the forces at play helps build awareness to make targeted, informed changes. Let's discuss your diet and how even little shifts can make a powerful difference.

The Domino Effect: From Your Plate to Your Nerves

Imagine each meal, no matter how large or small, as an event that either fosters or sabotages your blood sugar balance. It's NOT about perfection, but understanding the potential consequences of consistently putting the wrong building blocks into your body.

1. The Blood Sugar Spike

- **Rapid Digestion:** Refined carbs, sugars, and any processed food turn into glucose incredibly quickly. This isn't the same as the slow, steady fuel from complex veggies or whole-food sources. Think of it as a bonfire vs. a carefully controlled hearth providing lasting warmth.
- **Insulin Surges:** Your pancreas sends a signal of "all hands on deck" to try and bring order to this chaos. Insulin, a hormone, rushes in to shove that excess sugar into cells. In normal situations, this works, but chronically your system becomes overwhelmed.

2. Why Nerves Care About This Sudden Influx:

- **Energy Overload:** Nerves are metabolically active! Even a brief spike stresses their ability to produce energy efficiently, forcing them to rely on temporary backup systems that create oxidative damage long-term.
- **The Hunger Crash:** That quick dump of insulin often leads to blood sugar levels

bottoming out. This triggers cravings, shakiness, and mood swings, fueling a cycle of further bad food choices for fast "energy."

- **Inflammation Trigger**: Both the overload state AND the sudden plummet are inflammatory events. Low-grade constant inflammation is disastrous for delicate blood vessels critical to the health of your nerves.

3. The Neuropathy Connection

- **Overworked System**: Each time this roller coaster happens forces your body to adapt to manage the stress. This leads to insulin becoming less efficient, creating further risk, even when eating "reasonably" in the future.
- **It's NOT Just Diabetes**: Even small spikes within the "normal" lab range create damage if habitual. Over time this can lead to tingling, numbness, and altered sensation—all signs that your nerves are paying the metabolic price.
- **Cumulative Impact**: Each episode leaves a tiny trace of harm. Initially unnoticed, it adds up silently, increasing the risk of full-blown neuropathy. Worse, it leaves you vulnerable

to injuries and infections going undetected due to reduced sensation.

This is a simplified view, but understanding these steps makes dietary changes more than weight control–it's about preserving the health and function of your nervous system for the long run.

Fueling the Fire: Understanding Diet-Driven Inflammation & Oxidative Stress

Inflammation and oxidative stress sound like complex science. Yet, unhealthy food choices create a perfect storm for both processes to ravage delicate nerves, making simple dietary shifts incredibly powerful preventative medicine. Here's the breakdown:

1. Inflammation – Enemy of Nerves:

- **Not Just Red or Swollen:** Chronic low-grade inflammation is like a constant internal simmer. It disrupts every process. Think of this as your immune system on hyper-alert, reacting to diet like an invader, instead of doing its proper job.
- **Nerves Under Attack:** Inflammatory compounds released create irritation around nerves, reduce healthy blood flow, and weaken their outer protective layers. It's like

having a persistent chemical burn within your body.

- **Why This Matters:** Inflammation makes nerves hypersensitive and worsens ANY kind of neuropathy symptoms—burning, tingling, loss of feeling, you name it. It also hinders tissue repair if damage is already present.

2. Oxidative Stress: "Cellular Rust" That Harms Nerves

- **Metabolic Byproduct:** When unstable blood sugar and inflammation occur, our cells produce excessive "free radicals." Picture little rust bits damaging everything they touch. This happens everywhere, but your nerves are exceptionally vulnerable.
- **Attack on Tissues:** Oxidative stress causes cellular dysfunction, accelerates nerve deterioration, and hampers their natural "clean-up" process to remove waste. It's like a factory producing pollution instead of a useful product.
- **Reduced Protection:** Healthy fats and antioxidants fight this damage, but a poor diet lacks those defenses. Imagine sending firefighters equipped with buckets of water against a house fire fueled by gasoline.

3. The Cumulative Risk For Neuropathy

- **Silent for Years:** It can take time for all this to translate into neuropathy, but that damage never goes away. Unbalanced, inflammation-causing foods set the stage for far greater future vulnerability.
- **It Makes EVERYTHING Worse:** Even those genetically predisposed to neuropathy will see worse progression, pain resistant to typical treatment, and slower healing if inflammation and oxidative stress go unchecked.
- **Beyond Your Nerves:** High inflammation contributes to virtually every chronic disease, from heart problems to dementia. Addressing your diet yields body-wide benefits that influence many of your current (and future) health concerns.

The great news is this damage is REVERSIBLE. Strategic dietary changes and targeted support lower these firestorms, paving the way for healing and protecting your nervous system.

Building a House on Sand: How Dietary Choices Create Shaky Ground for Nerves

Imagine your nervous system as a complex interconnected web that requires specific raw materials for strength and the ideal environment to thrive. A poor diet does the opposite, creating a series of metabolic shifts that directly set the stage for neuropathy to take root.

1. The Blood Sugar Roller Coaster's Long-Term Toll

- **Insulin Resistance:** Constantly overloading your body with glucose-spiking foods means your insulin system becomes inefficient. It's like your cells stop responding to the doorbell! This is the beginning of what can escalate into diabetes.
- **Prediabetes:** Even mild, seemingly "normal" blood sugar elevations over time wear down your system. This silent process directly leads to nerve fiber damage, increasing the risk of full-blown neuropathy.
- **It's NOT Just About Symptoms:** Many people feel relatively fine and mistake this as a sign their diet isn't a problem. Lack of symptoms does not mean the underlying damage to nerves isn't progressing.

2. The Inflammation & Oxidative Stress Connection

- **Gut Health Impact:** Your microbiome (intestinal bacteria) thrives on diversity and healthy foods. A poor diet disrupts this balance. This leads to worsened inflammation and less absorption of the nutrients that your nerves rely on.
- **Toxic Burden:** Processed, chemically-laden foods overload your detoxification system. The buildup of toxins directly damages nerves. It also hinders your body's ability to produce the antioxidants needed to combat oxidative stress.
- **The Nutrient Gap:** Even if eating enough calories, a diet lacking diverse whole foods results in vitamin deficiencies. Without those vital cofactors, nerves can't function properly, no matter how hard they are trying.

3. Setting the Stage for Neuropathy

These factors don't mean you'll automatically become severely neuropathic, BUT they create conditions where:

- **Symptoms Appear Faster:** Even a genetic or situational predisposition to neuropathy will worsen exponentially faster in the toxic environment of poor blood sugar control and high inflammation.

- **Treatment Becomes Less Effective:** Addressing underlying causes is KEY to lasting nerve healing. If diet isn't tackled, medications or therapies only offer partial or temporary relief, while the root problem remains.
- **Overall Health Suffers:** Nerves aren't isolated! This dysfunction contributes to weight gain, metabolic diseases, and autoimmune flares, and lowers your resilience to other health challenges later in life.

The good news: It's NEVER too late to reverse course. Through targeted nutritional adjustments and support, we can create a pro-healing environment, stabilizing these processes and protecting both current and future nerve health.

Insulin: Your Blood Sugar Guardian (and How It Can Go Rogue)

Think of insulin as a key designed to unlock specific "doors" on your cells. When these doors open, glucose enters, providing energy for tasks from blinking to climbing stairs. In a healthy individual, insulin does its job efficiently, making sure that fuel is used or stored for later in a balanced way. Unfortunately, modern dietary factors and other underlying health conditions can make insulin less effective, or even turn it into an enemy for your nerves.

1. Insulin's Primary Tasks

- **Cellular Gateway:** Insulin signals specific cells – muscle, liver, fat – to transport glucose inside. Imagine your home requiring a key to get through the front door - glucose can't enter your cells without that insulin key.
- **Energy Regulation:** When it functions properly, insulin quickly lowers rising blood sugar levels after you eat. This protects you from the damaging spikes we discussed before.
- **Storage Manager:** When your immediate needs are met, excess glucose can be converted into glycogen under insulin's supervision. This is how your liver and muscles stockpile energy for later use.

2. When Insulin Plays A Role in Neuropathy

- **Overuse = Burnout:** Constant demand to shuttle away excess blood sugar due to poor diet leads to the cells 'tuning out' the signal insulin sends. They become insulin resistant, requiring a higher and higher amount to respond.

- **Uncontrolled Highs:** This overdemand on your pancreas (the organ that makes insulin) leads to exhaustion. If this progresses, your body becomes unable to even produce enough insulin anymore, leaving your blood sugar dangerously elevated.

- **Nerve Sensitivity:** Nerves have specific insulin receptors and are greatly impacted by imbalances. Even within 'normal' range blood sugar elevations, insulin spikes have both an immediate inflammatory effect and contribute to damage over time.

Important: Insulin itself isn't a bad guy. This intricate system allows cells to get the energy they need. The problem arises when this process becomes inefficient or overworked, ultimately affecting nerve health. Let's dive deeper into those concepts of insulin resistance and the importance of its counterpart, glucagon.

The Glucose Shuttle: How Insulin Directs Traffic and Why Nerves Pay the Toll

Imagine glucose like little energy packets circulating in your bloodstream after a meal. Insulin is the traffic cop directing these packets to their proper destination: your body's cells, where they can be used as fuel or stored for later. Nerves are highly metabolically active and rely on this constant energy source. Here's how problems arise:

1. How Insulin Helps Cells Take Up Glucose

- **Binding and Unlocking:** Insulin attaches to receptors on cell surfaces, acting as a signal to open specific channels (called GLUT4 transporters) to allow glucose entry. Think of a key working in a lock on a building's door.
- **Energy or Storage:** Once inside the cell, glucose has two possible fates. It can be used immediately for activities, or if there's enough for current needs, it can be converted into glycogen for a 'backup' supply later on.
- **Nerves & Insulin:** Your nerves are exquisitely sensitive to even subtle changes in insulin activity. They depend on that constant, steady delivery of glucose to maintain their metabolic function and repair processes.

2. The Neuropathy Link: When This Process Goes Awry

- **Insulin Resistance:** Cells become less sensitive to insulin's 'knock'. This means the key still works, but they require more and more of a signal to open and let glucose in. This leads to constantly elevated blood sugar levels.

- **"Hungry" Nerves:** While high circulating levels of glucose exist, your nerves (and other cells) are essentially starving because they cannot effectively access the energy. It's like having a full pantry but no way to open the door.

- **Direct and Indirect Damage:** High blood sugar levels themselves are toxic to nerves. Additionally, inefficient glucose uptake creates metabolic chaos within nerve cells, leading to inflammation and oxidative stress as covered earlier.

Important Note: Even if a person isn't diabetic, insulin resistance and chronically fluctuating blood sugar increase neuropathy risk significantly. This damage silently builds, with symptoms often not appearing until the process is well established and harder to reverse.

Understanding this allows us to look at interventions that not only treat neuropathy but focus on restoring healthy insulin function to protect your nerves long-term.

Glucagon: Your Blood Sugar Backup System

Think of your body's blood sugar regulation system as a carefully maintained dam with various gates controlling water flow. Insulin is one gate, letting excess 'water' in (glucose into cells) when levels are high. Glucagon is the gate that opens on the opposite side to allow stored reserves (glycogen) to be released when levels are too low, preventing your blood sugar from crashing. Neuropathy can occur with dysfunction on either side of this delicate balance.

1. Glucagon's Key Functions:

- **Stored Energy Access:** It primarily signals your liver to break down stored glycogen back into glucose. This steady trickle keeps blood sugar stable between meals and during fasting states like overnight sleep.
- **Prevents Dangerous Lows (Hypoglycemia):** In a healthy person, if you skip a meal, this mechanism kicks in to keep your body fueled. Severe lows are dangerous, but even minor dips can impact nerves negatively, as they require a constant energy supply.

- **Fat Metabolism:** Glucagon plays a supporting role in breaking down body fat for energy. This becomes extra important for those with insulin issues, as fat can be used as fuel when glucose uptake is dysfunctional.

2. The Neuropathy Connection:

- **Dysregulated Glucagon:** Unstable blood sugar due to poor diet and insulin resistance can also throw off glucagon production. Either excessive levels or an impaired response can contribute to neuropathy.
- **Blunted "Low" Signals:** In insulin resistance, even while blood sugar is still high, your body might mistakenly produce glucagon to release even MORE. This worsens the situation for your already struggling nerves.
- **Crash Risk:** As insulin dysfunction worsens, the risk of severe hypoglycemic episodes increases. While often considered a diabetes issue, even those with pre-diabetes can experience this dangerous drop, with negative consequences for their nerves.

3. Importance of Blood Sugar Balance:

Both high blood sugar and significant lows lead to nerve damage. While managing highs may seem the primary focus, supporting healthy glucagon function is essential for stabilizing this system. Nutritional strategies and targeted therapies can address this, restoring a more normal counterbalance to insulin action.

Finding Peace from Chaos: Insulin-Glucagon Balance Protects Nerves

Picture a complex dance between insulin and glucagon, a vital partnership keeping your blood sugar levels within a safe, narrow range. However, modern diet and lifestyle habits throw this elegant choreography into disarray. Chronic imbalance directly contributes to the metabolic distress that paves the way toward neuropathy. Let's delve into why this harmony matters and how it can be restored.

1. The Healthy Equilibrium

When functioning optimally, insulin and glucagon respond to your body's ever-changing needs. After a meal, insulin steps in to shuttle glucose efficiently into cells, ensuring adequate energy while preventing harmful blood sugar spikes. Hours later, or overnight, glucagon signals the release of stored energy, creating a steady, smooth stream of fuel for proper nerve function. Ideally, your blood sugar rises only modestly after eating and dips gently in between, all without your conscious effort.

2. When the Balance Breaks Down:

- **Persistent Highs:** Constant dietary overload forces insulin into overdrive. When cells eventually become resistant to its signal (insulin resistance), blood sugar levels remain continuously elevated. This bathes nerves in a toxic glucose solution.
- **Amplified Lows:** Even without severe hypoglycemia, blood sugar crashes trigger inflammation and stress responses within the nervous system. Chronic instability forces further glucagon dysfunction, increasing future crash risk in a downward spiral.
- **Metabolic Inflexibility:** Nerves thrive on a predictable, steady energy supply. Getting "stuck" with excess blood sugar they cannot access and then plummeting depletes them, weakens their defenses against damage, and impedes healing processes.

3. Protecting the Balance for Neuropathy Prevention

It's not about demonizing either hormone! True stability is found in supporting their intricate cooperation to handle fluctuating blood sugar within a narrow 'healthy' range. This involves addressing the root cause of insulin resistance through diet, optimizing natural glucagon production with specific nutritional strategies, and reducing stressors that disrupt both.

This approach fosters the ideal environment for your nerves, significantly reducing the risk of damage, and creates the perfect foundation for any other therapy to be even more effective at addressing existing neuropathy symptoms for long-term gain.

Beyond Blood Tests: Decoding the Early Signs of Insulin Trouble

Insulin dysfunction rarely happens overnight. It's a progression from healthy regulation toward cellular resistance and eventual burnout. Unfortunately, standard blood tests often miss these initial phases where intervention is most effective in protecting your nerves. Let's identify the telltale signs so you can take action early on.

1. Insulin Resistance at the Cellular Level

- **Reduced Sensitivity:** Cells become less responsive to insulin's signal, like a doorbell becoming faint. This means they take up less glucose from the blood, and your pancreas tries to compensate by pumping out more and more insulin.
- **The Neuropathy Link:** Even if blood sugar is still 'in range', nerves sense this shift. It creates a low-level hum of inflammation and inefficient energy production within nerve cells, setting the stage for future dysfunction and discomfort.
- **Silent Progression:** You can have significant insulin resistance and even pre-diabetic level blood sugars without noticeable symptoms for YEARS. Damage accrues under the radar, making prevention through lifestyle change essential.

2. Elevated Post-Meal Blood Sugar: A Warning Sign

- **The Spike and Crash:** Two hours after eating, healthy blood sugar should return to near baseline levels. If it remains high, it's a sign your insulin isn't efficiently lowering it. Even if fasting levels are good, this pattern is troubling.

- **Nerve Impact:** Even brief spikes damage delicate blood vessels, trigger inflammatory pathways, and create temporary metabolic 'blockades' within nerves themselves. Over time, this makes nerve fibers weaker and prone to the numbness/tingling characteristic of neuropathy.
- **It's NOT Just Desserts:** High-carb meals, especially processed ones, induce the most dramatic spikes. However, even 'healthy' carb loads can overwhelm an already taxed system if insulin is losing efficiency.

Spotting the Subtle Signs:

- **Energy Crashes After Eating:** Drowsiness, brain fog, and sudden hunger 2-3 hours after meals are signals your cells aren't getting enough glucose despite elevated blood levels.
- **Increased Belly Fat:** This type of fat signals insulin resistance, even if not overweight overall. It's due to your body storing excess glucose it can't efficiently push into cells.
- **Unexplained Skin Changes:** Random tags, dark patches (acanthosis nigricans), slow wound healing - these can reflect insulin dysfunction even without high blood tests.

Remember, the goal is to protect your nerves long-term! Recognizing these early patterns allows for dietary shifts and targeted support that prevent the progression of neuropathy.

The Tipping Point: Recognizing Moderate Insulin Resistance

At this stage, your body is constantly fighting to maintain blood sugar balance. While you may not have a diabetes diagnosis yet, internal metabolic chaos is wreaking havoc on your nerves. Understanding what's happening allows us to employ targeted strategies for reversal and protection.

1. Impaired Glucose Tolerance: The Bridge to Pre-Diabetes

- **Delayed Response:** After meals, your blood sugar rises higher and returns to baseline slower than ideal. This shows insulin isn't 'clearing' glucose efficiently – cells aren't listening to its signal effectively anymore.
- **Nerve Damage Underway:** Episodes of high blood sugar, even if followed by a drop, create inflammation, oxidative stress, and direct injury. Symptoms like tingling, sensitivity to

temperature, or mild numbness may appear sporadically.

- **Progression Risk:** Without action, this typically worsens into pre-diabetes. While this term sounds minor, the nerve damage happening in that state is NOT minor, and it becomes far harder to fully reverse the longer it goes on.

2. Metabolic Syndrome: A Perfect Storm for Neuropathy

This cluster of conditions is driven by insulin resistance and includes:

- **Belly Fat:** Not just about vanity, this visceral fat actively churns out inflammatory compounds directly impacting your nerves AND worsening insulin's ability to work.
- **High Blood Pressure:** Constricted blood vessels and disrupted circulation limit oxygen and nutrient delivery to your extremities, exacerbating any neuropathy symptoms.
- **Unhealthy Cholesterol Profile:** High LDL ('bad') plus low HDL ('good') leads to fatty build-up within blood vessels, further

compromising circulation your nerves depend on.

Why This Matters for YOUR Nerves

- **Combined Assault:** Each metabolic syndrome factor worsens the others, and all of them directly increase the rate of neuropathy damage. This isn't simply about future risk, but addressing this NOW prevents further, potentially irreversible injury.
- **Reduced Treatment Effectiveness:** Insulin resistance makes medications, supplements, and therapies meant to help neuropathy less effective. Tackling the root cause is essential for your program to have its intended impact.
- **It's NOT Inevitable:** This stage is a critical turning point. With knowledge and the right steps, you CAN halt the progression and reclaim metabolic health, safeguarding your nerve function for the future.

Let's discuss your situation and lab work so we can understand if you're in this moderate risk zone, and how to build a plan around addressing it.

The Crisis Stage: Severe Insulin Resistance and Your Nerves

Imagine your pancreas, responsible for insulin production, like a tireless worker on an assembly line. The constant demand for more and more insulin to address dietary overload leads to exhaustion. Cells tune out insulin's crucial signal, leaving your blood sugar uncontrolled. Without intervention, the impact on your nerves is severe and becomes exponentially harder to reverse.

1. Chronic High Blood Sugar: The Direct Assault on Nerves

- Beyond the Numbers: While often considered a diabetes issue, even "borderline" high blood sugars, sitting in the pre-diabetic range, cause significant nerve fiber damage over time if unaddressed.
- Cellular Chaos: When glucose saturates tissues, it leads to a cascade of destructive changes, including the formation of damaging byproducts (AGE products), hindering nerve function and repair ability.
- Worsening Symptoms: Neuropathy progresses more rapidly and is resistant to

typical treatment. Numbness, pain, balance issues, and complications like unrecognized infections become a major risk to your well-being.

2. Beta-Cell Burnout: A Vicious Cycle

- Loss of Insulin Production: The pancreas, overworked and under attack from inflammation, reaches its limit. Cells responsible for making insulin begin to fail, making blood sugar control nearly impossible without external help.
- The Progression to Diabetes: While a full-blown type 2 diabetes diagnosis may occur, neuropathy often appears before this diagnostic label. This doesn't mean your situation is less concerning.
- Exacerbated Nerve Damage: Inconsistent and uncontrolled blood sugars inflict the most severe harm. Nerves not only suffer from a lack of energy, but constant fluctuations create a chaotic environment where repair is stymied.

Crucial Note: This Stage Is NOT Inevitable!

Even here, strategic interventions can stabilize metabolic dysfunction, reduce inflammation, and support nerve health. While some damage may persist, we focus on preventing further rapid decline and improving quality of life. Here's the important distinction:

- **Without Action:** Neuropathy continues unchecked, leaving you increasingly vulnerable to falls, non-healing ulcers, and amputations. Systemic impacts worsen other health conditions or set the stage for them to develop.
- **With Informed Care:** We shift the trajectory. Even if some degree of blood sugar irregularity remains, supporting natural insulin function, reducing inflammation, and direct therapeutic support for your nerves make a world of difference.

The goal becomes maximizing function, minimizing complications, and fostering a resilient system that improves your outlook for the future.

Let's evaluate your personalized situation and find those crucial leverage points. With proper guidance and tailored support, you can still regain agency over your health and protect your nerves.

Let's shift our focus from blood sugar levels to the often-underappreciated concept of insulin fatigue and exhaustion. This process, driven by the constant overproduction of insulin, has insidious consequences for nerve health and sets the stage for neuropathy's development.

The Overworked Hormone: How Insulin Fatigue Sabotages Your Nerves

Picture insulin as a vital messenger, working tirelessly to maintain metabolic balance. However, chronic dietary demands can force it into overdrive, with long-lasting effects on your nerves even if your blood sugars haven't entered diabetic territory. Let's explore how this hidden dysfunction progresses and contributes directly to neuropathy risk:

1. Hyperinsulinemia: The Hidden Culprit

This term describes a situation where a seemingly normal fasting blood sugar masks a deeper issue - your body is flooded with chronically high insulin as it tries desperately to compensate for cells resisting its signal. Nerves are remarkably sensitive to insulin, making them a target of this dysfunction, long before a formal diabetes diagnosis.

Direct Nerve Injury: Excess insulin itself is inflammatory. Additionally, high levels paradoxically starve nerve cells by blocking effective glucose uptake. Over time, this combination damages delicate nerve fibers and impairs their ability to repair and transmit signals.

2. The Danger of Prolonged High Insulin

Even if blood sugar 'crashes' rectify the situation momentarily, the constant cycle of overproduction and resistance leaves several harmful consequences for your nerves:

- **Accelerated Damage:** Both high insulin states AND severe drops contribute to oxidative stress within nerve tissue, causing cellular harm that paves the way towards neuropathy's characteristic symptoms.
- **Insulin Resistance Progression:** The more overworked your system becomes, the faster it deteriorates. This makes it increasingly difficult to regulate blood sugar, even with drastic diet changes, worsening nerve health with each passing day.
- **Silent Progression:** Symptoms like tingling or numbness may be subtle or nonexistent

initially, lulling you into a false sense of security while damage silently builds in the background.

Recognizing the pattern: This insulin issue can be spotted through specific blood tests often overlooked in standard care. Symptoms suggestive of it include:

- Unexplained weight gain despite seemingly 'clean' eating
- Intense sugar cravings, especially after meals
- Difficulty losing weight despite exercise and calorie control

Understanding hyperinsulinemia allows for early intervention with targeted lifestyle shifts and support supplements that can break the cycle and PROTECT your nerves long-term.

Let's explore the downward spiral when overworked insulin production falters, culminating in beta-cell exhaustion and a profound acceleration of neuropathy progression and overall health decline.

Reaching the Breaking Point: Beta-Cell Failure and Nerves in Crisis

Your pancreas, the organ tasked with insulin production, initially tries valiantly to meet the unrelenting demand triggered by diet and insulin resistance. Yet, under constant bombardment from inflammation and metabolic stress, those specialized beta-cells tasked with creating insulin eventually falter. This transition is a crucial milestone in both neuropathy evolution and your overall metabolic health.

1. Beta-Cell Dysfunction: The Beginning of the End

- **Gradual Decline:** Beta-cells don't fail overnight. It's a progressive loss of both the quantity of insulin produced, and a disruption in the timing of when it's released in response to food intake.
- **Blunted "Peaks":** Healthy individuals get a sharp insulin spike after a meal to manage blood sugar. This weakens with dysfunction, leading to prolonged periods where glucose remains high, causing greater nerve damage than even consistent elevation.
- **Neuropathy Escalates:** Unpredictable fluctuations create a "double whammy" for your nerves. They not only lack a steady energy supply, but the swings trigger inflammation and disrupt vital repair processes they require for maintenance.

2. The Transition to Overt Diabetes

- **A Matter of Labels:** While a type 2 diabetes diagnosis is significant, it's useful to realize that metabolic damage and early neuropathy often predate blood sugars meeting the official threshold.

- **Amplified Damage:** In full-blown diabetes, beta-cell burnout leaves your body with little to no self-produced insulin. This leads to uncontrolled blood sugar spikes, further damaging vessels, worsening inflammation, and leaving your nerves deprived of vital protective nutrients.

- **Increased Complications:** Neuropathy progresses even with medications. The risk of wounds not healing, dangerous foot infections, and even amputations rises significantly. Managing the underlying cause is crucial, even with the best diabetic care.

Important Clarification: Insulin exhaustion doesn't mean your nerves are beyond help. Targeted therapies, addressing both nerve damage AND the metabolic drivers, become even more vital. Here's the distinction:

- **Without Focused Attention:** Neuropathy and other diabetes complications become more severe and difficult to treat, with devastating potential consequences on all aspects of your life and health.
- **With Informed Care:** We can stabilize the system to a degree, reduce harmful fluctuations, and support nerve health directly. This can positively impact symptoms, preserve function, and protect you from the worst-case scenario.

The goal is to preserve your quality of life to the fullest extent. Let's assess the precise stage of insulin dysfunction YOU are experiencing and create a plan centered around prevention and nerve function optimization.

The Unchecked Crisis: Consequences of Insulin Exhaustion for Neuropathy

When the body's ability to produce sufficient insulin wanes, it's as if the last line of defense against metabolic anarchy crumbles. Your nerves become caught in the crossfire, accelerating the damage and creating a cascade of complications. Here's how this plays out:

1. Uncontrolled Blood Sugar – A Perfect Storm for Nerves

- **Severe, Unpredictable Spikes:** With insufficient insulin, even modest meals send your blood glucose soaring. The longer it sits elevated, the more extensive the damage to fragile blood vessels and nerve fibers.
- **Lack of Fuel Supply:** Nerves starve even when drowning in a sea of unusable glucose. This cripples energy production, protective mechanisms, and the ability to transmit those vital signals needed for movement and sensation.
- **Oxidative "Rust":** Uncontrolled highs amplify oxidative stress, akin to internal rusting damaging cellular components within your nerves. This process weakens them irreparably, even if levels drop eventually.

2. The Threat of Neuropathic Complications

- **Progression and Resistance to Treatment:** Neuropathy intensifies, and even advanced therapies often fail to generate the same benefits when underlying metabolic chaos isn't simultaneously addressed.

- **Loss of Protective Sensation:** Numbness creates a high probability of injuries going unnoticed until they are infected and severe. Falls due to diminished balance become a major danger in daily life.
- **Circulatory Compromise:** Already damaged blood vessels suffer even more harm. Poor wound healing, particularly in the feet, becomes a constant concern and raises the specter of life-altering limb loss.
- **Systemic Breakdown:** Unmanaged blood sugars cause ripple effects. Heart disease, kidney failure, vision loss – all these risks dramatically increase, further hindering your body's ability to heal nerve damage.

Understanding the Stakes: This is meant to not instill fear, but to motivate towards action. Even at this stage, there are steps to improve stability and address complications directly! Here's how the outlook shifts:

- **Unmanaged:** Your neuropathy continues uncontrolled, with mounting disability, escalating risk, and a constant cycle of managing crisis situations that further erode your quality of life.

- **Action and Support:** You become an empowered partner in your care. We focus on calming the storm to the greatest degree possible, alongside direct nerve support. Goals become maximizing function, fostering independence, and safeguarding your overall health for the future.

This requires a comprehensive plan and may involve a team approach depending on the complexity of your case. Let's discuss your specific situation, and how, with informed action, we can chart a more empowered path toward managing your health.

Restoring Balance: Strategies to Safeguard Your Insulin Function and Protect Your Nerves

While the previous sections may feel heavy, here's the great news: insulin dysfunction and its impact on nerves don't have to be your inevitable future! Through targeted strategies, we can shift the trajectory towards better health, lessen neuropathy symptoms, and protect you long-term. Let's dive into the practical actions that empower you on this journey.

The Power of Your Plate: Dietary Strategies for Blood Sugar Balance

1. Rethink "Healthy" Carbs:

- Focus on Quality: Starchy vegetables, whole-grains in MODERATION, fruit paired with protein/healthy fats are all better choices than processed, refined grains. But even these will spike blood sugar significantly if the portion and combination isn't right for YOU.
- Individual Tolerance is Key: This isn't one-size-fits-all. We must uncover where your insulin system falters – is it big breakfast bowls of oatmeal, or even seemingly "low carb" sweet potato that causes issues?

2. The Importance of Protein and Fat:

- Slow and Steady Wins the Race: These nutrients help avoid rapid blood sugar spikes and crashes. With each meal, include quality sources like eggs, fish, nuts/seeds, avocado, and olive oil.
- Satisfaction Factor: Balancing macronutrients reduces those frustrating cravings that sabotage good intentions. This

creates sustainable change enjoyable for the long haul.

3. Not Just WHAT You Eat But WHEN:

- Timing Matters: Long overnight fasts, or skipping meals followed by large feasts worsen insulin resistance. Consistent, smaller meals may be better if you're prone to this.
- Mindful Snacking: Options like protein shakes or a handful of nuts between main meals can prevent energy crashes fueling poor choices later and help stabilize blood sugar.

Lifestyle as Medicine: Habits That Matter for Neuropathy

1. Movement for Metabolic Health:

- Type is Key: It's not just about burning calories! Resistance training, even brief bursts, improve insulin sensitivity dramatically. We will tailor activity to your fitness level and preferences
- Beyond the Gym: NEAT (Non-Exercise Activity Thermogenesis) counts! Daily walks,

standing more, even fidgeting increase sensitivity and provide nerve-specific benefits.

2. Stress: The Hidden Saboteur:

- Cortisol Connection: This stress hormone directly spikes blood sugar and worsens insulin resistance. Techniques to lessen the daily burden are non-negotiable!
- It's Not Just Mental: Undiagnosed gut issues, poor sleep, etc., are all physical stressors. A holistic approach uncovers all the triggers contributing to your metabolic stress load.

Important Note: This is an overview. Your individual path needs fine-tuning! We work together to assess your baseline and build achievable changes that will have the most significant impact.

Going Beyond Symptom Control: Functional Medicine for Neuropathy Risk

True healing goes beyond masking pain or simply managing blood sugar numbers. Functional medicine provides sophisticated tools for pinpointing hidden metabolic imbalances, nutritional deficiencies, and underlying inflammation contributing to your neuropathy risk or existing damage. Here's a glimpse at what this approach offers:

1. Targeted Testing - Uncovering What Conventional Labs Miss

- **Beyond Routine Panels:** HbA1c (3-month average blood sugar) shows PART of the picture. Tests like fasting insulin, oral glucose tolerance, or C-peptide provide clues crucial to understanding the stage of insulin dysfunction impacting YOU.
- **Inflammation Markers:** Highly sensitive CRP (hs-CRP), homocysteine, etc., show low-grade inflammation damaging nerves and worsening insulin resistance beyond what basic tests catch.
- **Nutritional Deficiencies:** Often, specific vitamin or mineral insufficiencies exacerbate neuropathy directly. Blood levels don't always reflect what's going on within your cells!

2. Addressing Root Causes, Not Just Numbers:

- **Autoimmunity:** Undiagnosed Hashimoto's (common!) attacking nerves may be present even if thyroid lab work seems "normal." Testing for these antibodies is critical if risk factors exist.

- **Hidden Gut Dysfunctions:** Leaky gut, SIBO, and poor digestion lead to inflammation and poor absorption of vital nerve-protective nutrients. Stool studies and other diagnostics are often needed to pinpoint specific issues.
- **Metabolic Individuality:** Genes, toxin load, and unique stressors influence how your body REGULATES blood sugar. This analysis goes beyond what's too "high" or "low" on a generic chart.

3. Personalized Therapies: Support That Goes Deeper

- **Targeted Supplementation:** Correcting deficiencies, and using specific nutrients proven to enhance insulin sensitivity, improve nerve-cell energy, etc., create a foundation for success.
- **Innovative Treatment Options:** Depending on the drivers of your neuropathy, therapies like nutrient-based IVs, photobiomodulation, or specialized modalities can accelerate healing alongside lifestyle changes.

- **Addressing the WHOLE Person:** Restoring optimal sleep, helping you develop a personalized movement plan tailored for your nerves, and working collaboratively with other providers you already see are crucial components of comprehensive care.

This approach yields information unavailable elsewhere, allowing us to design a roadmap for reducing neuropathy risk or maximizing healing potential far beyond generic advice.

Your Roadmap to Nerve Health: The Power of Individualized Neuropathy Care

There is no "one-size-fits-all" answer when it comes to protecting your nerves and lessening neuropathy risk. Your specific metabolic fingerprint, combined with your unique health history and current circumstances, necessitates a plan built around YOU. Let's explore why this is vital for lasting results.

Beyond Blood Sugar – Uncovering Your Story

- **Genetic Predisposition:** Some people are more prone to insulin resistance. Family history provides clues to the degree of urgency or specific areas we need to focus on aggressively for prevention.

- **Medical Background:** Past infections (like Lyme), medication use, and chronic conditions directly impact how we approach nerve support and blood sugar stability, as these can influence what therapies are both safe and effective.
- **Lifestyle Impact:** Shift work, high stress levels, and personal dietary habits all influence our starting point and what interventions will be sustainable, ensuring success as opposed to short-term changes that backfire.

The Importance of the "N of 1" Approach

This means treating you as a unique individual, not simply a cluster of symptoms. We use a combination of approaches to ensure this:

- **Progressive Assessment:** We may start with a few targeted changes as we gather data. Blood sugar monitoring with a meter, food logs, and symptom trackers give real-time feedback on what's working.
- **Tailored Testing:** Based on your initial intake, additional labs or diagnostics are often needed to address a lurking suspicion and personalize therapy,

ensuring we aren't wasting time with guesswork.

- **Dynamic Plan:** As your body responds and shifts, we adjust along the way. This could mean an increased focus on supporting restful sleep instead of just diet if that becomes a roadblock to progress, ensuring success!

Success Stories: Inspiration From Those Who've Triumphed

- The Prediabetic With Hidden Nerve Damage: A 52-year-old with 'borderline' high blood sugars dismissed fatigue until numbness started. Targeted support reversed this progression, saving them from severe complications.
- Finding the Hidden Trigger: A seemingly health-conscious woman in her 40s battled weight gain despite 'doing everything right.' Uncovering a gut issue led to finally achieving blood sugar control and weight goals!
- Beyond Just Numbness: Stress-driven insulin resistance worsened a patient's neuropathy

AND their chronic migraines. By calming the metabolic storm, both conditions improved simultaneously, something often missed.

These are just glimpses! Your success story is waiting to be written. Through partnership and a commitment to understanding YOUR body, we unlock the path to feeling better.

ACTION STEP: Insulin-glucagon balance is essential for maintaining healthy blood sugar levels. When this balance is disrupted, it can lead to many health problems, including neuropathy.

See if your blood sugar levels are higher than the normal range. If it's high, then we must get it under control to have a good chance of reversing neuropathy symptoms.

We will test fasting blood glucose and HbA1c. If you are interested in having your blood glucose level tested scan the code below.

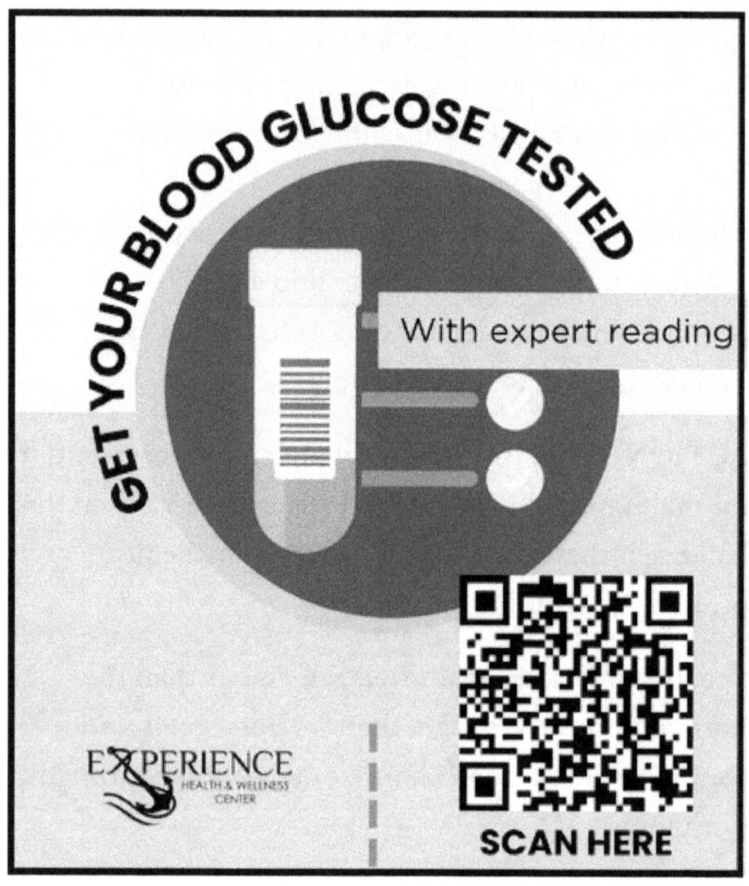

Unlock Your Path to Neuropathy Relief Now: Dial (239) 374-8654 to Speak With Us Today!

Kathleen: Rediscovering her 'Normal'

"I had lived with aches and pains for so long it had become my normal. Now, after six months, I am pain-free and no longer take daily doses of ibuprofen. Taking that initial

step and signing up for a consultation was the best decision I ever made!"

** Individual outcomes may differ.*

5

———

NOURISH, MOVE, DE-STRESS: RECLAIM YOUR NERVES

Nutrition: Your Nerves' Best Ally (or Foe)

Think of your nerves like a complex network of wires carrying messages throughout your body. Just as quality wiring is crucial for electrical systems, your nerves require specific nutrients to stay strong, repair themselves, and communicate properly. Diet directly influences these building blocks!

Why Your Food Choices Impact Neuropathy

- **Blood Sugar's Influence:** We've covered this previously, but reiterate how unstable levels damage nerves, especially those tiny blood vessels critical to nourishment. Diet is the first line of defense in managing this.

- **Nutrient Powerhouses:** Beyond simple calories, many foods contain compounds that protect nerves from inflammation, boost regeneration, and even improve signal transmission.
- **Toxicity Factor:** Processed, chemically-laden foods burden your detox system. With nerves already vulnerable, this added stress weakens them further and hampers the body's natural healing abilities.

Examples: Seeing the Direct Link

- **The Hidden Sugar Bomb:** That seemingly healthy smoothie or protein bar can contain as much blood sugar impact as a pastry. This triggers inflammation, making your nerves hypersensitive and less able to recover.
- **The Deficiency Trap:** Even eating 'well' doesn't guarantee enough of the B vitamins, magnesium, and antioxidants nerves crave. This leaves them unable to function optimally, even if medications temporarily mask the symptoms.
- **Good Fats Gone Bad:** Overconsumption of rancid cooking oils, processed meats, and fried foods generate harmful compounds that

literally damage the outer protective layer of nerve cells.

Remember: This isn't about blaming yourself – it's about understanding. Making targeted shifts can create both immediate and long-term improvements in nerve health.

The Investment in Your Nerves – Understanding the Costs and Benefits of Dietary Change

Shifting your diet isn't always easy. It requires breaking old habits and potentially trying new things. However, it's essential to understand this is an investment that impacts far more than just what you put on your plate.

Costs (Beyond Just Money)

- **Initial Effort:** Learning what foods work for your body and adjusting cooking methods takes time and energy. This can feel overwhelming at the start, especially alongside dealing with neuropathy symptoms
- **Social Changes:** Eating differently from friends and family can create challenges in some situations. Planning ahead helps prevent this feeling like a constant sacrifice!

- **Temptation:** Processed foods are designed to be addictive! Saying no becomes easier with time, but initially can feel like an uphill battle. Support is crucial here.

Benefits (Far Beyond Symptom Relief)

- **Independence:** Reducing your reliance on medications, managing conditions that worsen neuropathy (like uncontrolled blood sugar), and preventing falls or injuries through improved strength – these all translate to greater freedom and less reliance on others.
- **True Energy:** Stable blood sugar eliminates crashes and improves overall vitality. This means more capacity to do things you ENJOY, not just manage your illness.
- **Improved Health Beyond Your Nerves:** The same changes protect your heart, brain, and reduce your future risk of countless chronic diseases. This is a gift to both yourself and those you love!
- **Mental Boost:** Feeling in control of your health, knowing you're actively taking steps to improve, builds resilience and counters the

feelings of helplessness common with neuropathy.

Actions to Get You Started

1. **Find YOUR "Why":** Is it avoiding medication increases? Being able to play with grandkids? Whatever motivates you deeply, make that your fuel when changes are hard.

2. **Support is Key:** Partnering with our team ensures you're making the RIGHT changes for your situation and have accountability to create lasting habits, not temporary fixes.

3. **One Step at a Time:** Focus on adding in protective foods (plenty of veggies!) before completely restricting, creating less overwhelm. Progress, not perfection, yields success!

Let's discuss which costs you anticipate being most challenging, and how to ensure the benefits outweigh them - making this a sustainable, joyful shift for a better future!

Now we'll demystify the role of physical therapy and exercise for neuropathy. It's about WAY more than simply getting stronger. Here's how movement becomes medicine for your nerves.

Movement as Medicine: How Physical Activity Transforms Neuropathy

When neuropathy causes pain, numbness, or weakness, being active may seem like the last thing you want to do. Yet targeted movement, often under the guidance of a knowledgeable physical therapist, is a cornerstone of effective treatment and future protection.

Why Exercise Helps Your Nerves

- **Improved Circulation:** Well-planned movement encourages healthy blood flow. Those tiny vessels serving your nerves become more efficient, bringing in oxygen and nutrients while removing waste products.
- **Nerve Signal Boost:** Specific exercises can actually retrain how your brain and nerves communicate! This improves balance, and coordination, and lessens that 'disconnected' feeling common with neuropathy.
- **Muscle Matters:** Even with nerve damage, strengthening supporting muscles reduces strain and protects you from injury. This translates to greater daily ease of movement

and a lowered risk of further nerve damage due to falls!

- **Reduced Pain Signals:** Proper exercise has been shown to calm overactive pain signaling systems within the nerves themselves. This doesn't negate all discomfort, but can make it far more manageable.

Examples: Exercise for Neuropathy Goes Beyond the Gym

- **Aquatic Therapy:** For those with severe pain, exercise in water reduces the force of gravity, allowing movement with less stress on joints and nerves. This is often a confidence-building starting point.
- **Balance Retraining:** It's not just about not falling! Improving your sense of balance retrains the nervous system and helps counteract the distorted nerve signals causing numbness or instability in daily life.
- **Sensory Work:** Specific exercises designed around improving your sense of touch and awareness of where your body is in space directly influence how your brain interprets those faulty nerve signals.

- **Flexibility:** Tight muscles and fascia worsen nerve compression issues. Targeted stretching tailored for neuropathy alongside exercise makes other interventions even more beneficial.

This isn't about pushing through pain. Finding the right kind of movement, at a level appropriate for where you are NOW, is what yields long-term improvements in nerve health and quality of life.

Weighing the Effort vs. Reward

Similar to diet, initiating a movement plan requires investment. Let's look realistically at the potential costs, while emphasizing the immense benefits that go beyond just the physical symptoms of neuropathy.

Costs: Finding the Right Fit

- **Expense:** While often covered by insurance, co-pays and choosing a provider specializing in neuropathy can be costly. Consider if investing upfront saves in the long run due to needing fewer medications or avoiding future injury.
- **Initial Soreness:** Starting slowly is key, but some increased discomfort at first is normal

as your body adapts. Be honest with your therapist, but don't assume this pain means it's not working!

- **Accessibility & Time:** Finding a convenient location, and fitting sessions into your schedule may take logistical effort. View this as akin to important doctor appointments – an investment in your health worth the hassle.
- **"Not Seeing Results Fast Enough":** Nerve regeneration is slow. Small victories matter! Improved sleep after activity, a bit less instability on uneven ground – celebrate these even if the big goal of less pain takes longer.

Benefits: Transforming Your Life, Not Just Your Neuropathy

- **Improved Safety:** Better muscle tone, balance, and reduced falls directly lower your risk of a life-changing injury from a serious fall that further damages nerves. This is about true independence!
- **Functional Gains:** Tasks like opening jars, climbing a few stairs, or walking without

feeling unsteady become easier. This allows you to participate more fully in your daily life and not rely as heavily on others.

- **Pain Control:** While exercise isn't a magic fix for all types of nerve pain, it gives you a tool alongside other treatments, allowing you to become less medication dependent.
- **Empowered Mindset:** Knowing you're actively fighting back against neuropathy's progression lessens anxiety. Even on rough days, you have a sense of agency over your body, which is profound!

Actions for Success

1. **Honesty is Key:** Candid communication about your struggles with your therapist ensures the program is adjusted to help you see those benefits, making it worth the upfront effort.
2. **At-Home Habits:** Even on days without formal therapy, brief, nerve-focused movements boost results. Ask about a few things you can do for 5 minutes daily to make progress faster.
3. **Track the Wins:** Beyond pain scale changes, note things like, "Washed dishes without

dropping anything" or "Walked dog an extra block." This motivates you when progress feels slow.

Let's discuss which concerns you most about incorporating movement, so we find the way to make it sustainable and rewarding for you.

Calming the Storm: How Stress Management Impacts Your Nerves

Modern life is inundated with stressors, and if you're dealing with neuropathy, this burden can feel even heavier. Surprisingly, addressing stress levels is essential for your nerves to improve. Let's unravel the science behind this connection.

The Stress-Neuropathy Cycle

- **Fight or Flight Overrides Healing:** When your body perceives stress (even emotional, not just physical), it shunts resources away from processes deemed 'non-essential' like repairing nerve tissue.
- **Cortisol's Impact:** This stress hormone directly spikes blood sugar, even without eating. Nerves already vulnerable to these

fluctuations are hit even harder, worsening inflammation within the fibers themselves.

- **Pain Amplification:** Stress makes your nervous system hypersensitive. Even mild discomfort from neuropathy can become debilitating under constant internal 'alert' mode.
- **It's a Vicious Cycle:** Neuropathy pain itself is a major stressor, fueling the fire. Many techniques calm the nervous system on the spot AND have lasting impact, breaking this cycle for good!

Examples: How Stress Shows Up Disguised as Neuropathy

- **Worsening Symptoms Before "Big" Events:** Even joyful ones, like a trip, can increase flare-ups as your body anticipates demand beyond the usual routine.
- **Sundays Are the Worst:** For many, the dread of returning to a stressful job manifests physically with worsened nerve symptoms, hindering your ability to rest.
- **Trouble Sleeping Despite Exhaustion:** Dysregulated stress hormones make your

brain feel wired even when your body needs rest. This further depletes your resources for nerve healing.

- **Digestive Distress:** The gut-brain connection is potent! Stress impacts things like motility and the microbiome, indirectly making neuropathy worse through disrupted absorption and increased body-wide inflammation.

Important: Stress isn't a character flaw! This is how the nervous system evolved for survival. The problem is, chronic modern stress never turns OFF, impacting you on a cellular level.

Stress Relief: An Investment with Priceless Returns for Your Nerves

Prioritizing stress management might feel like one more thing to add to your already full plate. Yet, understand that this is NOT about bubble baths and scented candles (though those can be nice!). It's about finding targeted practices that shift your nervous system's baseline, yielding benefits that ripple throughout your entire health journey.

Costs: It Takes Effort

- **Learning Curve:** Mindfulness techniques, or breathing practices, take time to master enough to reap benefits. Early on, it can be frustrating with your mind wandering constantly - this is normal!
- **Carving Out Time:** Even brief practices done consistently are best. This may initially feel like you're stealing time away from other responsibilities, adding to your stress load.
- **May Uncover Deeper Issues:** Effective stress work often brings up unresolved emotional burdens or past traumas. While a sign of progress, this requires support and a willingness to seek help if needed.

Benefits: Transforming Your Response to Both Neuropathy and Life

- **Resilience Boost:** You gain tools to handle unavoidable stressors, like a bad symptom flare, without it completely unraveling you. This improves quality of life dramatically.
- **Less Pain Sensitivity:** Techniques like deep breathing directly impact the pain signaling centers within the nervous system. It doesn't cure neuropathy, but it makes it far more tolerable.

- **Blood Sugar Factor:** Effective stress management reduces cortisol spikes, helping stabilize blood sugar. This takes pressure off your nerves and makes any other dietary efforts more impactful.
- **The Ripple Effect:** Improved sleep, better digestion, and a greater sense of calm have benefits for every aspect of your health beyond neuropathy, creating positive momentum towards overall well-being.

Actions to Make it a Habit

1. **Start Small:** Designate even just five minutes at the same time daily for a guided breathing exercise or mindfulness app. Consistency matters more than long practices sporadically.
2. **Track Progress Beyond Symptoms:** Note things like, "Handled an argument calmly" or "Fell asleep quickly despite the pain." This shows you the power this has over your entire experience, not just temporary relief.
3. **Enlist Support:** If you notice practice stirs up unresolved stress, don't ignore it! Finding the appropriate therapist or support group

makes this deeper healing possible, which has a lasting impact on your nerves too.

Let's explore which simple stress reduction techniques resonate with you so we can create a doable starting point and ensure this becomes an empowering part of your overall treatment plan.

Beyond Conventional Care: The Power of Integrative Medicine for Neuropathy

Integrative medicine takes a whole-person approach. It acknowledges that while necessary, traditional neuropathy treatments often fall short, leaving patients feeling frustrated. This approach examines all factors contributing to your unique case and employs evidence-based therapies alongside medication for a more comprehensive plan.

Why Consider an Integrative Approach?

- **Finding the Missing Pieces:** Sophisticated testing helps uncover issues often overlooked, like nutrient deficiencies that make nerves sluggish, or hidden gut disturbances fueling inflammation that worsens your symptoms.

- **Root Cause Focused:** Instead of simply chasing symptoms, we target the drivers of damage. For example, if autoimmune processes are attacking nerves, managing this is vital, not just numbing the pain.
- **Personalized Treatment Options:** There's no single 'alternative cure' for neuropathy. A skilled practitioner tailors innovative therapies based on YOUR body's needs, increasing the chances of meaningful results.
- **Enhancing Existing Treatment:** Integrative strategies often make medications work better and reduce the need for harsh dosages. It's a truly collaborative approach aimed at maximizing your outcome.

Examples: Integrative Therapies for Neuropathy

- **Targeted Nutrient Support:** Beyond basic vitamins, this may encompass high-dose delivery (like a B12 injection), or specific compounds shown to calm inflamed nerves or support regeneration.
- **Advanced Healing Modalities:** Techniques like laser therapy, specialized electrical stimulation, or biofeedback can accelerate

nerve repair beyond what's possible with just diet change and standard rehab alone.

- **Personalized Botanicals:** Certain carefully chosen herbs and plant extracts have scientific backing for improving nerve function, blood vessel health, and reducing pain signals when used under professional guidance.
- **Gut-Neuropathy Connection:** Restoring microbiome balance, healing leaky gut, and addressing infections like SIBO can significantly impact neuropathy, even when digestive symptoms aren't your primary complaint.

Important Note: Collaboration is essential. Finding a practitioner trained in safely integrating these approaches with your medications and established protocol is key.

Let's discuss if pursuing an expanded approach feels helpful or overwhelming. Often, even a few targeted interventions alongside established care can make a big difference.

Weighing the Potential: Understanding the Costs & Benefits of Integrative Medicine

Incorporating integrative approaches means venturing beyond familiar territory. It's wise to consider the potential investment and rewards to decide if this path is right for your neuropathy care.

Costs: A Different Way of Thinking

- **Financial:** Advanced testing, specialized therapies, or custom supplements may not be insurance-covered. It's essential to be transparent about your budget when working with a provider to prioritize the most impactful choices.
- **Time Commitment:** A thorough initial intake, more frequent follow-ups at first, and the potential trial of various therapies require patience and commitment to the process. Results aren't usually as immediate as with medication.
- **Mindset Shift:** This approach requires being open to strategies outside the conventional model. A willingness to explore the interconnectedness of your health is key to unlocking root-cause solutions.
- **Potential Frustration:** Not every therapy will be a magic bullet. However, each one provides more information, refining your

treatment plan and increasing the likelihood of long-term success.

Benefits: Expanding Your Path Towards Healing

- **Uncovering Hidden Roadblocks:** Identifying an untreated thyroid issue, vitamin deficiency, or inflammatory trigger fueling your neuropathy can bring relief when other treatments seem to stall
- **Enhanced Outcomes:** Many integrative strategies, like specialized nutrient combinations, make physical therapy more effective or improve your blood sugar control far better than diet alone.
- **Reduced Medication Reliance:** While often still necessary, the goal is minimizing side effects by targeting the cause. This improves the quality of life, even if neuropathy can't be fully eradicated.
- **Hope and Empowerment:** Knowing you're leaving no stone unturned in pursuit of better health builds a sense of resilience, crucial when dealing with any chronic illness.

Actions for Informed Decisions

1. **Vet Providers Carefully:** Look for certifications relevant to neuropathy and integrative treatment, and ask about their success rates working with similar cases to yours.

2. **Start with One Area:** If the idea feels daunting, focus on a single aspect, like gut health testing or considering a specific nutrient therapy alongside your current plan. Small initial wins build confidence!

3. **Honesty About Budget:** Discuss financial concerns openly with a potential provider. Many offer tiered programs or can suggest ways to prioritize the highest-impact items within your means.

Let's talk about which aspects of an integrative approach intrigue you most, and which feel concerning. We can find ways to explore options that balance potential benefits with the realities of time and financial investment.

This chapter has outlined the ways nutrition, movement, and stress management directly impact your neuropathy. Don't underestimate the power you hold to influence your own healing.

As Brittney discovered: "If I could give Dr. Omar 50 stars, I would. Before I was recommended to their office, I had constant numbness in my arms and hands on a daily basis. After seeing Dr. Omar, I no longer have any numbness, and I feel like I have a new body. He truly is a master of his craft!"

** Your results may be different.*

Remember, this journey isn't just about managing symptoms, it's about reclaiming your life. You deserve to feel like you have a 'new body', and with the right approach, that can become your reality too.

ACTION STEP: Get Your Neuropathy Relief Stretch Handbook. Master 11 Key Stretches from Home To Retrain Your Nerves and Regain Your Life.

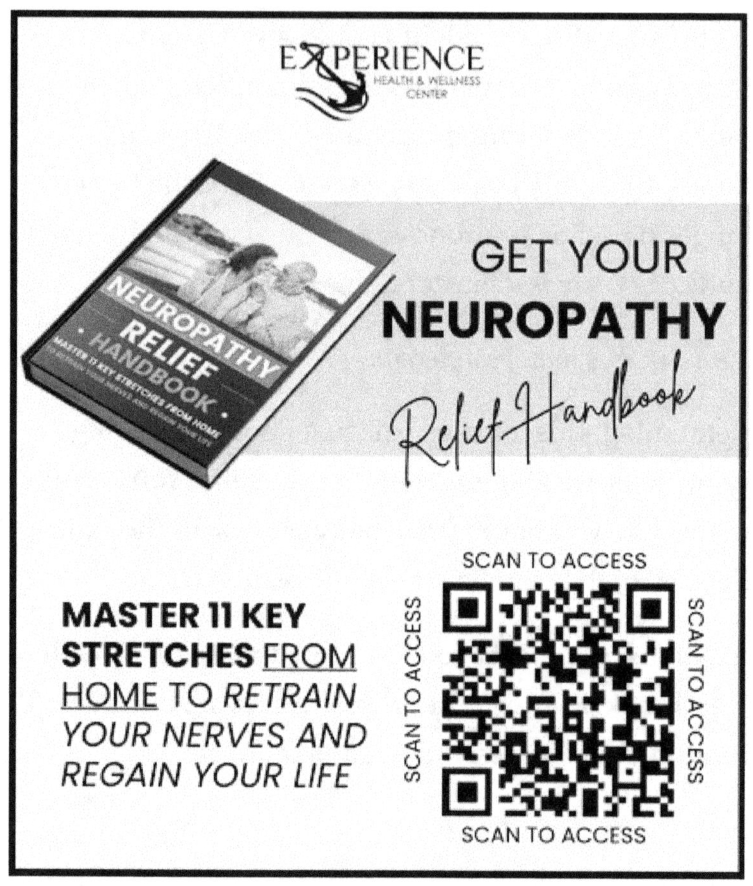

Unlock Your Path to Neuropathy Relief Now: Dial (239) 374-8654 to Speak With Us Today!

6

UNVEILING THE R.E.S.T.O.R.E. NEUROPATHY PROGRAM

The phone call came on a Tuesday, the voice on the other end hesitant yet hopeful. "Dr. Clark," a man named Peter began, "I've heard about your program, but... well, I've tried so many things. Will this really be different?" Peter had been struggling with neuropathy for years, the numbness and tingling in his hands making even simple tasks like buttoning a shirt feel impossible. He'd been told it was just a part of aging, something he'd have to learn to live with.

Peter's story wasn't unique. So many individuals fighting neuropathy feel lost in a maze of treatments that offer little lasting relief. That's why I created the R.E.S.T.O.R.E. program – a roadmap to guide them back to health.

When Peter came in for his initial evaluation, it was clear conventional approaches had failed to address the root causes of his neuropathy. Blood sugar imbalances, a vitamin B12 deficiency, and even a subtle spinal misalignment were all contributing to his nerve dysfunction.

Over the next few months, we worked together, implementing personalized dietary changes, targeted supplementation, and gentle chiropractic adjustments to improve nerve communication. Slowly, Peter began to feel the difference. The numbness lessened, his grip strength improved, and a sense of hope replaced his initial skepticism. Peter's journey wasn't about a magical overnight cure, but about uncovering the specific issues driving his neuropathy and addressing them with precision. It was about empowering him to become an active participant in his own healing.

It's important to remember that Peter's experience is his own and may not reflect typical results. Individual outcomes with the R.E.S.T.O.R.E. program can vary depending on a variety of factors.

Peter's story underscores the core principle of this chapter. It's a collaborative process where we work together, as a team, to pinpoint the unique factors contributing to your neuropathy and create a personalized plan to address them. It's about taking control, understanding your body's needs, and embracing the possibility of a brighter, healthier future.

For many, neuropathy feels like a cruel twist of fate, something happening TO you without a clear reason. However, the R.E.S.T.O.R.E. Neuropathy Program hinges on understanding that lifestyle factors significantly influence the severity of symptoms and the potential for healing. It's NOT about blame, but about giving you powerful tools to reclaim control over your own health.

The Power of Choice: How Lifestyle Influences Your Nerves

- **Beyond Just Symptoms:** Diet, movement patterns, stress levels – these all DIRECTLY impact the underlying processes driving neuropathy, not just how bad things feel.
- **Metabolic Control:** Unstable blood sugar and inflammation damage delicate blood vessels that nourish nerves AND hinder your body's inherent repair abilities.
- **Nerve Communication:** Physical activity enhances circulation and boosts nerve

signaling. Conversely, inactivity worsens numbness and pain sensitivity long-term.

- **The Stress Factor:** Constant stress elevates harmful hormones and depletes your body of resources critical for nerve regeneration and balanced function.

Giving Examples: Seeing the Connections

- **The Hidden Sugar Hit:** That "healthy smoothie" spikes blood sugar more than a pastry, making your nerves hypersensitive and less able to recover from injury.
- **Desk Job Danger:** Sitting for hours, even with exercise, worsens circulation. This means less oxygen and nutrients reach your nerves, hindering healing.
- **Sleep Struggles:** Stress-driven insomnia disrupts nerve repair processes. Even with adequate daytime rest, nerve signals stay out of sync, amplifying pain.

Explaining the Costs & Benefits

- **Costs:** These changes aren't always easy initially – adjusting habits takes effort, and there will be slip-ups. Support is crucial for turning this into a win!

- **Benefits:** The payoff is HUGE. By stabilizing blood sugar, moving strategically, and reducing stress, you lessen the damage nerves endure daily AND make treatments more effective.

Actions: Making It Real

- **Food & Mood Journal:** Not about calorie counting, but noticing patterns. Do 'healthy' meals leave you crashing, making nerves act up hours later? Does stress make you crave sugar? This data is your roadmap.
- **Movement Audit:** Track daily activity, even small stuff. Spot patterns – worse on days you don't even walk the dog? Find simple ways to boost baseline movement.
- **Stress Triggers:** Identify when those overwhelming feelings start. Work commute? Arguments with a loved one? This isn't about fixing those, but having QUICK tools to calm your system when they happen.

This information is POWER. Let's dive deeper to understand your specific starting point, so those first steps on your RESTORE journey create results you FEEL fast!

Now let's illuminate the cornerstone of the RESTORE program: pinpointing the unique drivers of YOUR neuropathy to ensure those efforts are maximizing your potential for healing.

Unmasking the Enemy: Targeted Testing for Neuropathy Root Causes

Think of standard medical care as focusing on extinguishing a raging fire - suppressing the immediate symptoms. Root cause discovery is about finding the source of the sparks that keep reigniting it. This unlocks a plan designed specifically for you, giving you a better chance at long-term relief. Here's how:

Going Beyond Basic Labs: Your True Health Fingerprint

- **Inadequate Standard Testing:** Blood sugar checks and basics like B12 often come back "normal" even with significant issues contributing to your neuropathy. This creates frustration and fuels the feeling treatment is a guessing game.

- **Metabolic Deep Dive:** Tests like fasting insulin, oral glucose tolerance, or comprehensive inflammatory markers tell us HOW your body is handling blood sugar – the primary fuel your nerves need.
- **Hidden Contributors:** Gut health issues, micronutrient insufficiencies, thyroid dysfunction impacting how you USE fuel – uncovering these allows us to support your body's inherent healing capabilities instead of just fighting symptoms.

Examples: Not Just Numbers, But Clues

- **"Borderline" Blood Sugar:** Often dismissed, even slight elevation matters for fragile nerves. Targeted dietary changes may be more impactful than medication if caught early.
- **Low-End "Normal" Vitamins:** Levels just within ranges might not be enough to promote optimal nerve repair. Supplements tailored to YOUR results are more effective than generic ones.
- **Unexplained Gut Issues:** Even if not your main problem, bloating, etc., indicates inflammation. This fuels neuropathy and

hinders the absorption of nutrients key to nerve health.

Costs & Benefits of Expanded Testing

- **Costs:** May not be fully covered by insurance. It's worth exploring, as this often yields MORE savings by preventing wasted money on ineffective therapies long-term.
- **Benefits:** Reduced frustration! Knowing WHY you respond differently to treatment than someone else empowers both you and your practitioner.
- **Personalized Plan:** Test results inform the type of diet, the ideal level of physical activity, even which stress-reduction techniques are likely to have the greatest impact on your nerves – NOT one-size-fits-all.

Actions: Collaborate for Results

- **Ask Questions:** Don't accept, "All your labs are fine" without seeing copies! Understanding your numbers is crucial for advocating for further testing.
- **Prioritize:** If finances are tight, we can focus on areas most likely contributing based on

your case. Often, even a few targeted tests change the plan's efficacy dramatically.

- **Connect the Dots:** Bring in results from past tests, no matter how old. Tracking trends helps see the big picture, especially when you've noticed symptom shifts over time.

Ready to be your own health detective? Let's examine the clues your body is providing. This knowledge will guide your RESTORE program toward maximizing those obtainable outcomes.

Breaking the Cycle: Removing Roadblocks to Neuropathy Healing

With a map of your unique root causes in hand, we now take decisive action to dismantle the forces fueling your neuropathy! Think of it as clearing overgrown weeds so the delicate new growth of healing has room to flourish. This involves targeted strategies, both addressing what's directly harming nerves AND supporting your body's inherent ability to clean up past damage.

Targeting the Culprits: Protecting Your Nerves from Further Harm

Based on YOUR test results, we target any ongoing contributors to imbalanced blood sugar, elevated inflammation, or other issues impacting nerve function. Think of this as putting out those lingering sparks within your system. This can include:

- **Strategic Dietary Shifts:** Not just generic "eat healthier" advice. This involves adjusting meal composition, timing, and specific foods to stabilize blood sugar in the way YOUR body needs.

- **Addressing the Gut Connection:** Treating infections like SIBO, balancing gut bacteria, and healing leaky gut have profound benefits for neuropathy by reducing systemic inflammation and nutrient malabsorption.

- **Metabolic Support:** Targeted supplements may be necessary to correct deficiencies revealed in testing. This is not always needed long-term but is often a kickstart to the healing process.

Examples: What This Looks Like in Action

- **Hidden Gluten Sensitivity:** Even without Celiac, this triggers inflammation in many. A trial elimination can be a game-changer, and we work to ensure it's balanced for nerve-nourishing nutrients.

- **Finding Your Sugar Triggers:** It may be processed junk food, OR seemingly healthy choices your body doesn't tolerate as well. Blood sugar monitoring gives us real-time feedback.
- **Beyond Diet:** If stress keeps cortisol surging, the best diet in the world won't be enough. Tools specifically suited to YOUR triggers are essential alongside those changes.

Costs and Benefits of Targeted Action

- **Cost:** Honesty is key. Thorough gut protocols or supplements can be an investment, but often are what prevent needing harsher meds down the line.
- **Benefit:** Confidence! Knowing you're addressing what's driving your neuropathy makes healthy habits stick because you feel the impact it has on your symptoms.
- **Ripple Effect:** These same changes often improve sleep, energy, mood – making this a total transformation, not just a begrudging sacrifice to lessen foot pain.

Actions: Building Sustainability

- **No Perfection Needed:** Small wins matter! Even partial adherence can yield benefits, allowing us to fine-tune what works realistically for YOUR life.
- **Food Focus:** Plan ahead to reduce reliance on hasty choices. A few staples to grab instead of hitting the drive-thru are powerful.
- **Support is Key:** Partners, helpful apps, or a like-minded group aid accountability. This shouldn't feel isolating, even when YOUR needs are different from others.

Let's break down your results and determine those high-impact starting points. Remember, removing these obstacles allows the rest of the RESTORE plan to work even better, giving you the best chance to achieve those transformative outcomes.

Beyond Just Numbing: Advanced Tech for Targeted Neuropathy Relief

Neuropathy pain is notoriously complex. While essential, medications often leave you feeling foggy or provide incomplete relief. These cutting-edge therapies target your unique pain patterns while boosting your body's own healing response – offering a multi-pronged approach to finding greater comfort.

Harnessing the Power of Modern Science – Tools to Quiet the Storm

These therapies directly impact nerve signaling, repair processes, and circulation – they aren't just a temporary distraction from discomfort. Options include:

- **Specialized Electrical Stimulation:** Different frequencies can calm overactive pain receptors, increase blood flow to damaged fibers, and even encourage regrowth of small nerves.
- **Photobiomodulation (Laser Therapy):** Specific wavelengths of light energy reduce inflammation, stimulate repair within the nerve, and can improve sensation in numb areas over time.
- **Frequency Specific Microcurrent (FSM):** This subtle therapy works to re-balance distorted nerve signals and is customizable based on your primary symptom type (burning, pins and needles, etc.)

Examples: When Tech Provides the Missing Piece

- **Stubborn Localized Pain:** Even with lifestyle changes, a specific area may remain hypersensitive. Targeted laser to that zone can significantly improve comfort for day-to-day function.
- **Stabilizing Sleep:** Calming nerve pain with FSM often leads to better sleep. This gives your body vital recovery time, and indirectly impacts how you feel throughout the day.
- **Enhancing Other Treatments:** Often, tech plus a lower medication dose provides better control than either alone. This lessens potential medication side effects long-term.

Costs & Benefits: An Investment in Recovery

- **Cost:** May not be insurance-covered. It's vital to discuss your budget upfront to prioritize those most likely to help, and if rentals vs. purchasing makes sense.
- **Benefit:** True relief means greater ability to work, be active, and engage socially – this has quality-of-life benefits tough to quantify, alongside the physical improvement.

- **Not a Magic Wand:** These therapies work best within a comprehensive plan. When combined with the RESTORE program, they often accelerate progress, yielding deeper and more lasting effects.

Actions: Exploring Your Options

- **Research Matters:** Reputable providers will happily explain the science behind the tech, tailored to YOUR neuropathy type (diabetic is different than post-injury, etc.).
- **Ask About Trial Sessions:** Some clinics offer this. Don't expect miracles right away, but it helps determine if it shows promise before greater investment
- **Be an Informed Partner:** Tracking your symptoms before/after each type helps us fine-tune the approach for your unique response. This avoids wasting time on ineffective options.

Let's discuss your biggest pain struggles. Often, even a temporary reduction with tech boosts motivation to keep strengthening healthy habits, fostering a positive cycle.

Igniting Your Inner Healer: Strategies to Optimize Nerve Recovery

Your body has a remarkable ability to mend itself, but neuropathy creates conditions that hinder this process. Through targeted nutrition, specialized supplementation, and other supportive therapies, we create an environment where your system can focus on restoration, not just fighting to survive!

Harnessing the Power of Nutrients for Nerve Regeneration

- **Beyond Basic Vitamins:** While a good multivitamin is important, specific nutrients have proven benefits for regenerating damaged nerves, reducing inflammation within fibers, and improving nerve signal transmission.
- **It's About Synergy:** These nutrients work together! Targeted blends tailored to neuropathy are far more effective than increasing a single compound on your own.
- **Food First, Then Fill the Gaps:** Dietary shifts are vital, but even when eating well, absorption issues or individual needs might mean targeted support is the missing puzzle piece.

Examples: Nutrients That Can Make a Difference

- **Acetyl-L-Carnitine:** This powerful antioxidant protects against cellular damage, especially within nerves, and may promote new fiber growth after injury.
- **Alpha Lipoic Acid:** Helps improve nutrient delivery to damaged nerves and reduce oxidative stress, a major contributor to neuropathy pain.
- **High-Dose B Vitamins:** The forms matter! Specialized types are easier for your body to USE for repair, crucial when those systems are compromised.

Costs & Benefits: Investing in Restoration

- **Costs:** High-quality, bioavailable supplements can be a financial investment. Discuss this openly with your provider to prioritize the most impactful ones within your budget.
- **Benefits:** Reduced Inflammation = Less Pain! Often, this allows lower doses of pain medication for better control without the side effects.

- **Protecting Your Future:** Healing on a cellular level makes you less prone to flare-ups and may slow the progression of neuropathy overall.

Actions to Maximize Success

- **Timing Matters:** Some nutrients work best on an empty stomach, others with food. Following dosing guidelines ensures proper absorption and maximum effect.
- **Watch for Interactions:** Discuss ALL medications/supplements with your doctor. Even natural therapies can sometimes interfere with prescription drugs.
- **Listen to Your Body:** Not everyone tolerates all supplements well initially. We may need to gradually increase dosages or try different delivery methods (liquid vs. capsule) for optimal results.

Let's review your current diet and any supplements you're taking. We can optimize your intake with the dual purpose of reducing current symptoms while empowering those long-term healing mechanisms.

Upgrade Your Daily Habits: Lifestyle as a Superpower for Neuropathy

You've likely heard about the importance of diet, exercise, and stress for overall health. But in the RESTORE program, we harness these daily actions as targeted therapy for your nerves. Small, sustainable shifts, tailored to your unique situation, accumulate powerful benefits over time.

Building a Foundation for Healing: Optimizing the Basics

This isn't a generic list of "shoulds." Our focus is on personalized tweaks that create the MOST positive impact on your neuropathy. Key areas include:

- **Nourishing Your Nerves:** Meal timing, balancing healthy fats and protein, and strategies to keep blood sugar stable based on YOUR individual responses are paramount.
- **Movement Matters:** Finding the right type, at the right intensity for your current fitness level, is vital. This improves circulation AND nerve signaling, not just overall well-being.
- **Sleep Sanctuary:** Restorative sleep is when nerve repair processes kick into high gear. We

identify what's disrupting yours and build habits for better quality and quantity of sleep.

- **Mindful of Stress:** Even short bursts of techniques to downregulate your nervous system throughout the day accumulate a huge impact on pain perception and halting neuropathy's progression.

Examples: Personalized Lifestyle Support

- **The Breakfast Debate:** For some, skipping it entirely steadies blood sugar. For others, a specific type prevents a midday crash that worsens nerve pain. We figure out what's YOUR ideal pattern.
- **Beyond the Gym:** Short walks after meals, targeted stretches at your desk – these might have greater nerve benefits than exhausting workouts that leave you too sore to continue consistently.
- **Tiny Stress Tamers:** Deep breathing app notifications, changing your stressful commute to a scenic route – finding small ways to inject calm into the chaos matters for long-term resilience.

Costs & Benefits: It's an Investment, Not a Sacrifice

- **Change Is Hard:** Be honest about what feels overwhelming! Small steps are better than grand plans that lead to abandoning it all. Support is key!
- **Benefits Go Beyond Your Feet:** Improved sleep, mood, energy levels, etc., are spillover effects that make the whole process feel worthwhile, even when nerves themselves heal slowly.
- **Protecting Your Future:** These habits are preventative medicine for your WHOLE body, reducing your risk of many chronic illnesses that become more dangerous when neuropathy is present.

Actions: Where to Start

- **Pick ONE Area:** Diet, sleep, adding in brief movement – what feels most achievable right now? Focus yields early wins, motivating further change down the road.
- **Track the Wins:** "Walked 10 mins without worsening pain" is as important as any scale change! This highlights the benefit and keeps you going when progress feels slow.

- **Find Your Tribe:** A walking buddy, an online forum of others focusing on healthy habits, even just a supportive partner – connection helps you stay accountable on difficult days.

Let's determine those small tweaks most likely to yield big improvements for YOUR neuropathy. We will prioritize enjoyment and sustainability alongside effectiveness, for a lifestyle transformation that empowers you for the long haul.

Protecting Your Gains: Strategies for Long-Term Neuropathy Success & Well-being

The RESTORE program isn't about a quick fix, but a transformation into sustainable health. This final stage is crucial. We build a personalized maintenance plan and address mindset shifts to keep you empowered long after those initial victories.

Prevention-Focused Aftercare & Ongoing Support

Neuropathy can progress or flare despite healthy habits. This is NOT a failure, but means we adjust the plan proactively, so setbacks are minor, not a slide back to where you began. This includes:

- **Long-Term Monitoring:** Periodic retesting, symptom trackers you keep at home, etc., help catch subtle changes early and tweak the plan before things worsen significantly.
- **Maintenance Protocols:** These might be abbreviated versions of therapies you found helpful in active treatment, lower dose supplements, or specific check-ins to address stressors before they fuel symptom flares.
- **Continued Learning:** As research evolves, or your life circumstances change, new tools or strategies become available. Staying engaged in your care keeps you empowered to implement the best options for YOU.

Examples: Preventing "Backslides"

- **Travel Troubles:** A fun trip shouldn't undo months of work! We develop strategies to maintain healthy choices on the go, addressing the usual pitfalls you've encountered in the past.
- **The "Flare-up Toolkit":** If pain worsens, instead of panic, you have a pre-approved plan to quickly address it. This could be a temporary med increase, targeted home

therapies, etc. – knowing there's action to take lessens the anxiety that fuels the problem.

- **Honest About Stress:** Big life events happen. Proactive tools honed in the initial phases, and ongoing support, help navigate these without your nerves paying the price long-term.

Costs & Benefits: Investing in Lasting Wellness

- **Cost:** Maintenance might mean occasional therapy sessions, test expenses, etc. Preventing hospitalization or the need for stronger meds often balances this out financially.
- **Benefit:** Reduced Fear & Uncertainty! Knowing you have a plan and support reduces the stress that worsens neuropathy. This has a profound impact on ALL aspects of your health.
- **True Freedom:** It's not about constant vigilance, but building habits and skills that become second nature. This frees up mental energy to live your best life, not obsess over your health.

Actions: Creating Your Personalized Plan

- **Identify Your Triggers:** Do specific foods, stress, less sleep always coincide with worsened symptoms? These are our red flags for focused early intervention in the future.
- **What Support Looks Ideal to YOU:** Is it check-ins every 6 months? Being part of an online community? This is as important to long-term success as any diet change!
- **Celebrate Milestones:** Mark on your calendar 3-month, 6-month, etc., anniversaries of starting this journey. Reflect on what's better, not just how far there's still to go.

This phase should feel empowering, not another burden. Let's create a roadmap that preserves the progress you've worked so hard for, ensuring those outcomes you achieved with RESTORE give you the best life possible – one where neuropathy is a manageable part of your story, not the whole plot!

ACTION STEP: Scan the code below to download our 25 Anti-Inflammatory Recipes Guide.

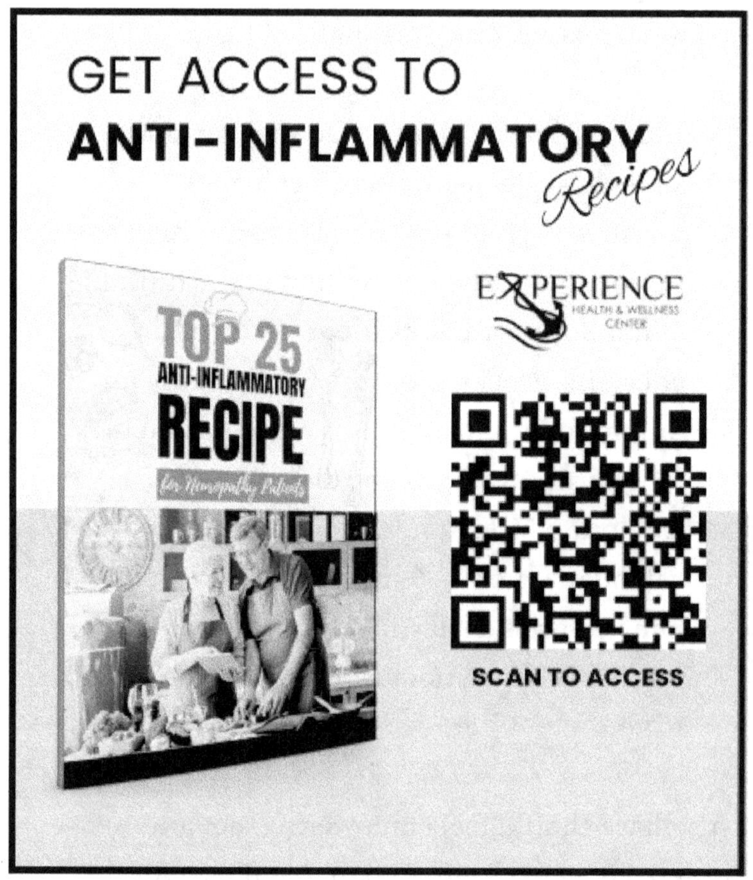

Unlock Your Path to Neuropathy Relief Now: Dial (239) 374-8654 to Speak With Us Today!

7

———

YOUR PATH TO HEALING: DISCOVER THE R.E.S.T.O.R.E. SOLUTION

Throughout this journey, we've explored the complex ways neuropathy impacts your life and how conventional treatments often fall short of providing lasting relief. Now, it's time to unveil the comprehensive RESTORE Solution. This isn't just about masking symptoms. It's a framework for unlocking your body's inherent healing potential and fostering lasting well-being.

Embracing the RESTORE Methodology: Your Roadmap to Recovery

The RESTORE method stands apart by systematically addressing the interconnected factors fueling your neuropathy through personalized strategies designed to:

- **Regenerate Damaged Tissue & Nerves**
- Enhance Circulation
- Stimulate Nerve Fibers
- Tried & True Methods
- Obtainable Outcomes
- Restore Balance
- Elevate Your Life

Think of it like tending a garden. We don't just yank at weeds (your symptoms). We provide nutrient-rich soil (targeted support), ensure proper sunlight and water (lifestyle), and give those delicate seedlings (your nerves) time to flourish again.

Examples: How RESTORE Makes a Difference

- **Persistent Pain Despite "Good" Blood Sugar:** Addressing gut health alongside diet can lead to better nutrient absorption, reducing inflammation that makes nerves hypersensitive.
- **Exhausted by Therapy:** Finding the right kind of movement INCREASES energy, allowing you to reap the full benefit of other treatments and feel better in daily life.

- **Isolated & Afraid:** A support system helps you navigate setbacks, reminding you they are temporary, and celebrating success beyond just a change in test results!

Costs & Benefits: An Investment in Your Future Self

- **Costs:** Commitment to change is essential – new routines take effort initially. Specialized testing or therapies may have out-of-pocket costs we discuss transparently.
- **Benefits:**
    - Less reliance on medication and its side effects
    - Improved overall health reducing other medical costs down the road
    - Regaining independence and joy in activities you thought were lost to neuropathy
    - The confidence of knowing you're doing EVERYTHING possible to create a brighter future!

Actions: Start Your RESTORE Journey

1. **Reflect on Your "Why":** What specific

outcome do you dream of? Hold onto this when the path feels challenging.

2. **One Step at a Time:** Choose ONE area from our previous exploration (diet, stress, etc.) where you feel ready for change.

3. **Track It:** Not just numbers! Journal how changing that ONE thing impacts how you feel, both good and bad. This data is as powerful as any lab test!

Let's dive deeper into each principle of RESTORE, creating a personalized plan, so those initial small steps lead to significant and sustained improvement. Call us at (239) 374-8654 or visit our website, efchealth.com/neuropathy, to schedule a neuropathy evaluation today.

"When I went to the consultation, I was really not very hopeful of anything happening positively. And it turned out what they were going to do was so different from what I had seen before. As I went and started using the process, I never varied. I stayed with it the whole time, and it worked. I got my feeling back." - Stan

** This is one individual's experience and does not guarantee similar results.*

Going Beyond the Standard: Why R.E.S.T.O.R.E. Offers a Unique Solution

If you're frustrated by feeling like neuropathy treatment is a never-ending cycle of medications with harsh side effects, yet minimal symptom relief, you're not alone. The RESTORE method isn't a rejection of conventional care, but an expansion beyond it. It fills the critical gaps, increasing the potential for meaningful, long-lasting improvement in your quality of life.

Root Causes vs. Symptoms: The Key Difference

- **Traditional Focus:** Often revolves around medications designed to numb pain signals, control blood sugar, or calm irritated nerves. While necessary for many, this leaves the WHY behind your neuropathy unaddressed.
- **RESTORE Approach:** We certainly focus on symptom relief, but also prioritize uncovering:
    - Hidden blood sugar instability, even if tests were "normal"
    - Specific nutrient deficiencies making nerves sluggish
    - Unmanaged stress fueling both

inflammation and making you
hypersensitive to pain
  ○ Gut health problems impacting your
    WHOLE system, not just digestion
- **It's a Partnership:** RESTORE encourages
  collaboration with your current providers,
  optimizing their care by targeting what's
  often not considered in a standard medical
  model.

Examples: When Changing the Focus Changes the
Outcome

- **The Vitamin Mystery:** Despite medication,
  someone's numbness worsens. We discover
  low B12, but NOT deficiency-level. The right
  kind of supplementation dramatically
  improves their outcome!
- **Sleep Struggles:** Sleep medications help
  initially, but then stop. Targeted stress
  reduction techniques break the insomnia
  cycle, indirectly lessening pain due to better
  nerve repair overnight.
- **Stubborn Blood Sugar:** Standard diet advice
  fails to control spikes. Identifying food
  triggers unique to a patient finally gets things

stable, protecting nerves AND improving energy.

Costs & Benefits: Understanding the Trade-Off

- **Costs:** May involve additional testing, specialized therapies not always covered, and time commitment to implement changes.
- **Benefits:**
    - Less trial-and-error with medication or procedures that leave you feeling worse
    - Reduced long-term health costs, by preventing complications of uncontrolled neuropathy
    - Improved mood and energy, making treatment itself less of a burden
    - The empowerment of knowing you're TRULY doing everything for the best possible outcome

Actions: Questions to Guide Your Path

1. **Ask About Root Causes:** Don't assume the answer is "that's just neuropathy." Inquire about tests beyond the basics or factors your doctor may not have considered due to time limits.

2. **Track Medication Impact:** Are you getting significant symptom relief, or just tolerating harsher side effects? This data is valuable!

3. **Be Your Own Advocate:** Research reputable sources about the links between lifestyle and neuropathy. Come armed with questions, showing you're seeking a collaborative solution.

Let's discuss your experiences with conventional treatment. This pinpoints areas where the RESTORE method can add that missing piece to your treatment puzzle, ensuring results justify the effort it requires.

Building a New Normal: Weaving R.E.S.T.O.R.E. into Your Everyday

True healing isn't about a temporary, intense program that leaves you burnt out when it's over. The RESTORE method provides a pathway for integrating sustainable change. Think of it like gradually building strength and endurance – it takes consistent action, but the reward is being able to do more without exhausting yourself!

Small Shifts, Big Impact: The Power of Daily Choices

Integrating RESTORE means:

- **Prioritizing Nourishment:** Not about restrictive dieting, but building meals to optimize blood sugar stability and provide the building blocks your nerves crave.
- **Movement as Maintenance:** Finding activity you enjoy, at a level that supports circulation and nerve health without leading to painful flares.
- **Taming Everyday Stress:** Short, simple practices throughout your day to interrupt chronic "fight or flight" that hampers healing.
- **It's a Process:** Perfection isn't the goal! Small wins, tracked carefully, become the foundation you gradually build upon to create lasting habits.

Examples: What This Looks Like in Real Life

- **The Breakfast Switch:** Skipping it used to lead to cravings by lunch. A protein-rich smoothie now provides hours of steady energy and lessens afternoon nerve discomfort.
- **Lunchbreak Power:** A 10-minute walk around the block instead of eating at the desk

improves pain by evening, making after-work activities more enjoyable.

- **Phone Reminders:** Simple deep breathing app alerts break up the workday, cumulatively reducing the overall stress burden impacting sleep.

Costs & Benefits: It's an Investment, Not a Sacrifice

- **Costs:** May involve changing long-standing routines, which sometimes feels harder than expected. Support is key when ingrained habits fight back!
- **Benefits:**
  - Feeling in Control: Knowing your actions directly impact your well-being counters the helplessness neuropathy often brings.
  - Improved "Baseline": Even on bad days, you bounce back faster because you've strengthened your overall health foundation.
  - Ripple Effect: Better sleep, mood, energy, etc., aren't just a bonus! They make the hard work feel worth it, fueling your motivation for continued progress.

Actions: Start Where You Are

1. **Your Biggest Struggle:** Be honest! If cooking is daunting, ordering one healthy meal delivery service daily is a victory. Don't get overwhelmed with fixing everything at once.

2. **Hidden Time Pockets:** Track your phone use. Could just 5 minutes of scrolling become a walk once a day? Find where "mindless" activities can be swapped for health-focused ones.

3. **Accountability Matters:** A text buddy, app, or even a visible calendar with daily goals makes you far more likely to stick with it long-term.

Let's analyze your typical day. We will pinpoint those micro-moments ripe for RESTORE upgrades that feel achievable and build momentum toward becoming your strongest, most resilient self.

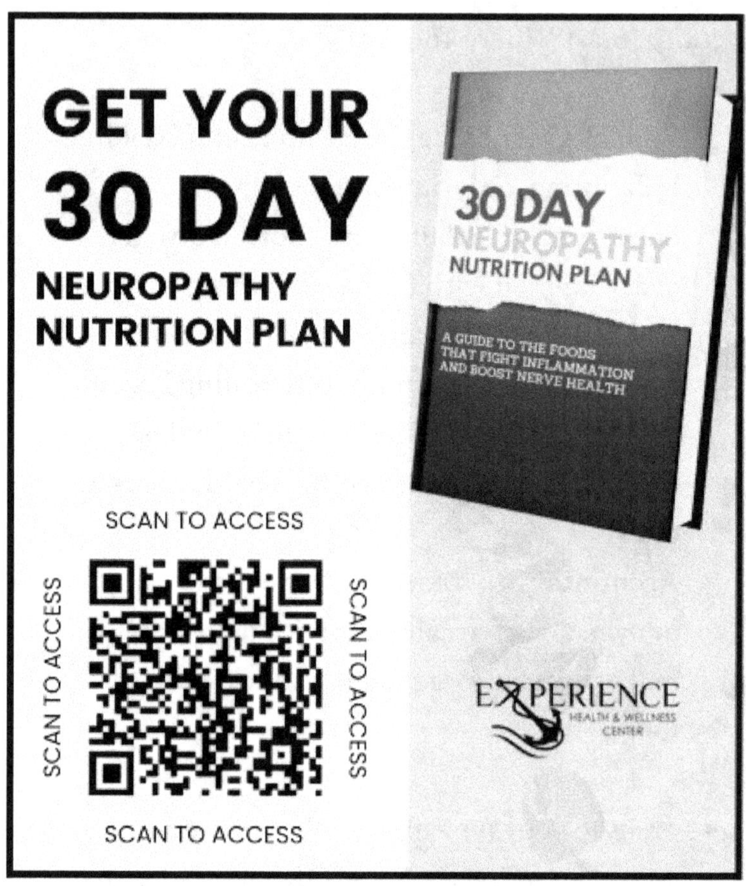

Unlock Your Path to Neuropathy Relief Now: Dial (239) 374-8654 to Speak With Us Today!

8

———

THE NERVOUS SYSTEM CENTRAL TO GOOD HEALTH

The look on Maria's face was one I'd seen countless times before: a mix of fear and frustration. "It's like my own body has turned against me," she confided, her voice trembling slightly. Maria had been diagnosed with an autoimmune disorder, and lately, she'd been experiencing strange, seemingly disconnected symptoms: bouts of dizziness, digestive issues, and a persistent tingling sensation in her feet. Her doctors struggled to explain it, attributing it to anxiety or simply the side effects of her medication.

But my intuition told me something else was at play. After a thorough examination and targeted testing, the pieces of the puzzle fell into place. Maria was experiencing autonomic neuropathy, a form of nerve

245

damage affecting the involuntary functions of her body. While her autoimmune condition was likely a contributing factor, years of chronic stress and poor gut health had further compromised her nervous system, creating a perfect storm for neuropathy to take root.

This chapter is about understanding this intricate and often overlooked network that controls every aspect of our well-being. It's about recognizing that nerve damage isn't just about numbness and tingling in the extremities; it can manifest in a wide range of seemingly unrelated symptoms, impacting everything from digestion to heart rate.

Maria's journey toward healing wasn't just about managing her autoimmune disorder; it was about supporting her entire nervous system. We implemented a multi-pronged approach that included gentle chiropractic adjustments to reduce nerve interference, stress-reduction techniques to calm her overactive nervous system, and dietary changes to nourish and repair damaged nerves.

Over time, Maria's symptoms began to subside. The dizziness lessened, her digestion improved, and the tingling in her feet became less frequent and intense. Most importantly, a sense of hope replaced her initial fear as she gained a deeper understanding of her own body and its remarkable ability to heal. Maria's story is a testament to the power of a holistic approach that recognizes the central role of the nervous system in overall health and well-being.

While Maria's story is inspiring, it's essential to understand that individual results can vary. This testimonial is not intended to represent typical outcomes, and not everyone will experience the same benefits. Every patient's journey with neuropathy is unique.

Think of your nervous system as a bustling metropolis, humming with electrical signals that control every aspect of your life. These nerve pathways are the messengers, ensuring your body functions seamlessly— from how you move and digest food to the steady rhythm of your heartbeat.

Neuropathy, however, disrupts this delicate communication. Imagine faulty telephone lines— messages get scrambled, leading to the frustrating symptoms associated with the condition. This disruption can throw off your balance, making simple walks a challenge. Digestion can become unpredictable, causing discomfort. Even your ability to get a restful night's sleep is often compromised as those misfiring nerves continue to send errant signals.

But here's where hope shines through: your body has a remarkable ability to heal. And that includes your nervous system. While neuropathy may feel overwhelming, the RESTORE approach is all about unlocking your potential for healing. It's about creating the perfect conditions for your nerves to regenerate, paving the way for a return to function and a life less burdened by pain.

Your Nervous System: A Simplified Look

Let's simplify the nervous system to understand how it's impacted by neuropathy. Think of it as having two major divisions:

1. **The Central Nervous System (CNS):** This is your mission control center, made up of your brain and spinal cord. It's where information is processed, thoughts form, and commands are sent throughout your body.
2. **The Peripheral Nervous System (PNS):** Picture this as a vast network of cables extending from your spinal cord, reaching every part of your body. It controls sensation (like touch and temperature), movement, and automatic functions like your heartbeat. This is the area neuropathy primarily affects.

A Closer Look at Your Nerves

Think of each nerve as a miniature communication cable. The core "wire" carrying the messages is the axon. Surrounding it is a protective layer called the myelin sheath, similar to the insulation around electrical wires.

Neuropathy can damage both the axon and its protective sheath. Damaged insulation leads to scrambled signals, causing those uncomfortable or painful sensations. Sometimes, the "wire" itself breaks down, leading to numbness and loss of feeling. These disruptions explain the challenging symptoms of neuropathy.

Neuropathy Explained: What Triggers Nerve Damage

Our nerves are remarkable structures, but unfortunately, they're also vulnerable to damage. This damage leads to neuropathy, which comes in a few different forms:

- **Peripheral Neuropathy:** Our primary focus, this occurs when nerves in your hands, arms, feet, and legs are compromised. This is what causes those frustrating sensations like pain, numbness, and tingling.

- **Autonomic Neuropathy:** This type impacts nerves that control your body's automatic functions, like digestion and heart rate. While less common than peripheral neuropathy, it's crucial to be aware of.

The Domino Effect of Neuropathy

Rarely is neuropathy caused by a single issue. Instead, it's often a chain reaction, with multiple factors contributing to nerve damage. Some of the major players include:

- **Unstable Blood Sugar:** Fluctuating blood sugar levels wreak havoc on your entire body, including your delicate nerves.
- **Inflammation:** Imagine a low-grade fire constantly smoldering within your body. Nerves are particularly sensitive to this inflammatory damage.
- **Nutritional Deficiencies:** Your nerves depend on specific nutrients to function properly and repair themselves. When your diet lacks these essentials, your nerve health suffers.

- **Other Medical Conditions:** Diabetes is a major risk factor, but neuropathy can also stem from other ailments like autoimmune disorders, thyroid problems, or even past infections or exposure to toxins.

Key Takeaway: Successfully conquering neuropathy requires more than just masking symptoms. The RESTORE approach focuses on uncovering and addressing the unique root causes driving your nerve damage, promoting true healing.

Neuroplasticity: The Key to Nerve Regeneration

There's incredibly good news for those struggling with neuropathy: your body possesses an amazing capacity to heal itself, even when it comes to your nerves. This is thanks to a remarkable phenomenon called neuroplasticity.

Think of neuroplasticity as your brain and nerves' ability to adapt, rewire, and forge new connections. It might take time, but this process lays the groundwork for lasting recovery from neuropathy.

How to Ignite the Healing Process

Here's how we can foster this natural healing:

- **Essential Nutrients:** Your nerves need a steady supply of B vitamins, magnesium, and other vital nutrients to repair and rebuild.
- **Lifestyle Changes:** Prioritizing restful sleep, managing stress, and engaging in appropriate movement reduce inflammation and create an optimal environment for nerve regeneration.
- **The RESTORE Approach:** Our program blends targeted therapies to stimulate nerve growth, boost blood flow, and calm inflammation. When combined with those nutrient and lifestyle shifts, remarkable healing becomes possible.

Patience & Persistence

Remember, healing is a journey, not a sprint. By recognizing and actively supporting your body's innate ability to heal, you pave the way for significant, long-term improvements in managing your neuropathy.

Stress & Neuropathy: The Hidden Link

Healing isn't just about addressing the physical roots of neuropathy. The connection between your mind and body plays a powerful role in how you experience and recover from this condition.

Stress: The Enemy Within

When you face a perceived threat, your body's "fight or flight" response kicks in. This ancient survival mechanism is designed for short bursts – think escaping a dangerous animal. However, chronic stress, a common issue in modern life, keeps you in a constant state of high alert.

This has ripple effects throughout your body. Stress hormones like cortisol flood your system. While useful in the short term, chronic elevation of these hormones fuels inflammation, a key driver of neuropathy pain. Plus, your blood pressure rises, and your immune system takes a hit.

The impact on neuropathy is twofold. First, heightened inflammation directly aggravates your nerves, making symptoms like pain, tingling, and numbness worse. Secondly, when your body is focused on managing constant stress, it has fewer resources to dedicate to healing those damaged nerves. It's like trying to fix a leaky roof while a hurricane is raging.

Stress Relief: Unlocking Recovery

Managing stress isn't merely about feeling calmer. It's essential for allowing your body to prioritize healing. Here are some techniques particularly beneficial for individuals with neuropathy:

- **Mindfulness Practices:** Simple exercises like focusing on your breath for a few minutes can ground you and quiet a racing mind.
- **Gentle Movement:** Forms like yoga, tai chi, or mindful walking ease tension while also improving circulation, a win-win for neuropathy!
- **Guided Relaxation:** Explore apps or recordings offering guided meditations to help you cultivate a state of deep relaxation.

Consistency is key. Incorporating even short stress-reduction practices into your daily routine can make a remarkable difference in your overall well-being and your journey with neuropathy.

The Power of Hope: Fueling Your Recovery

It's easy to dismiss the idea of a positive mindset as wishful thinking. But when battling neuropathy, your attitude can have a profound impact on your progress.

Breaking Free from Limiting Beliefs

If you convince yourself that you're trapped by neuropathy or that things will only worsen, those thoughts can become a self-fulfilling prophecy. By shifting your mindset to embrace the possibility of healing, you open yourself up to the full potential of the RESTORE program.

Mind Over Matter

You're right, a positive mindset isn't a magic cure for neuropathy. However, it can significantly influence your experience of the condition and your progress within the RESTORE framework. Here's how:

- **Taming Stress:** We've discussed how chronic stress wreaks havoc on your nervous system. A positive outlook helps you manage those inevitable stressful moments. This translates directly to lower inflammation levels, which can lead to reduced pain and improved nerve function
- **Unleashing Resilience:** Healing often isn't linear. Some days are easier than others. A positive mindset fuels your determination. It helps you bounce back from setbacks and stay committed to your treatment plan.

- **Embracing Possibility:** When you approach challenges with a "can-do" spirit, you're more open to trying new therapies and lifestyle modifications. This proactive attitude optimizes your chances of finding the strategies that make the biggest difference for your unique case.

Remember, your mind and body are deeply intertwined. When you shift your mindset for the better, you're creating a powerful ripple effect that supports your journey towards conquering neuropathy.

Hope: Your Constant Companion

Healing journeys are rarely predictable. There will be good days, and there will be days that feel more challenging. In those tough moments, hope is what keeps you moving forward.

Picture hope as a beacon of light. It illuminates the possibility of a better future, even when your current reality feels difficult. This deep-rooted belief in your body's potential to heal, combined with trust in the RESTORE process, fuels your determination.

When progress seems slow or you experience setbacks, hope reminds you that healing isn't always a straight line. It's that inner voice that tells you to keep going, try one more thing, and never give up on yourself.

Remember, even small victories are worth celebrating. Hope allows you to find joy in these milestones, sustaining your motivation and reinforcing your belief that a life with less pain and improved function is truly within reach.

Knowledge is Power

By now, you've gained a solid understanding of your nervous system and how neuropathy disrupts it. This knowledge is empowering because it shifts you from feeling like a victim of this condition to an active player in your own healing process.

A True Partnership

The RESTORE approach acknowledges the complexity of neuropathy. It goes beyond simply treating the physical symptoms. It addresses the mental, emotional, and lifestyle factors that influence your nervous system's health as a whole.

Repair, Rebalance, Renew

Think of your nerves as a communication system. Our program gives you the tools to repair damaged "wires," boost the signal strength, and teach your body healthier habits. This comprehensive approach sets RESTORE apart, maximizing your chances of lasting relief and a life less burdened by neuropathy.

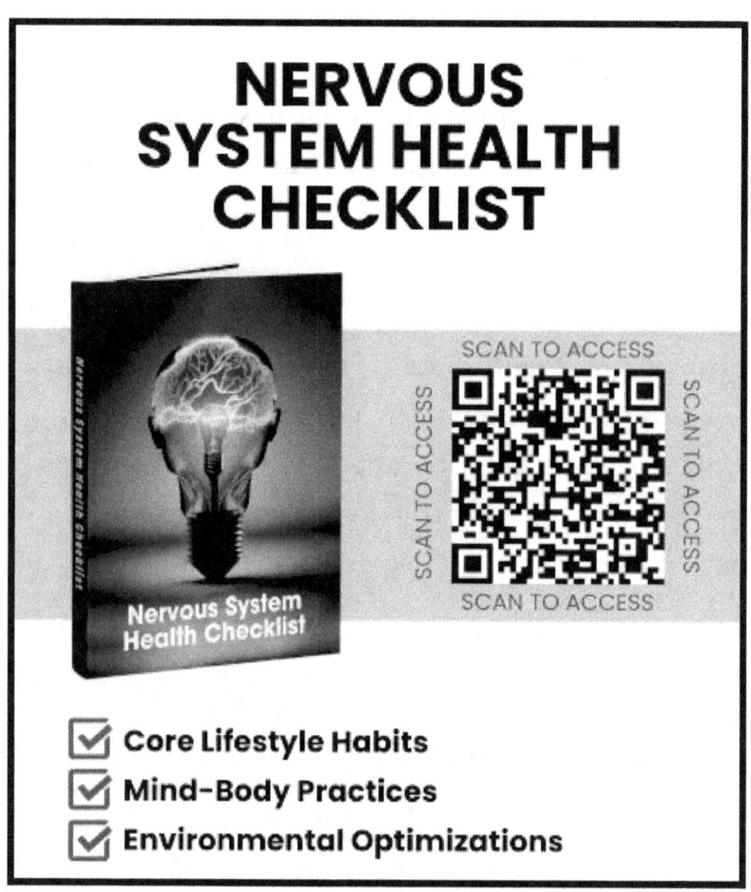

Unlock Your Path to Neuropathy Relief Now: Dial (239) 374-8654 to Speak With Us Today!

9

———

STATINS & NEUROPATHY: WHAT
YOU NEED TO KNOW

Jeremy, a man in his late 70s, sat across from me, his brow furrowed with worry. "My doctor says my cholesterol is too high," he explained, "and he wants me to start taking statins. But I'm already dealing with this neuropathy, and I'm afraid the medication will make it worse." Jeremy had heard the warnings about statins and nerve damage, and he was understandably hesitant.

Jeremy's concern was valid. Statins, while effective at lowering cholesterol, can have a detrimental impact on nerve health. These medications interfere with the production of CoQ10, a vital nutrient that powers your cells, especially your nerves. Depleting this crucial energy source can worsen existing neuropathy or even trigger new symptoms.

Chapter 9: Statins & Neuropathy: What You Need to Know is about empowering you with the knowledge to make informed decisions about your heart health without jeopardizing your nerves. It's about understanding the risks, exploring alternatives, and advocating for your well-being.

With Jeremy, we delved into his specific cardiovascular risks, carefully weighing them against the potential consequences of statin use. We implemented a comprehensive plan that focused on lifestyle changes, targeted supplementation, and addressing underlying factors contributing to both his high cholesterol and neuropathy.

Over time, Jeremy's cholesterol levels improved significantly without the need for statins. More importantly, his neuropathy symptoms stabilized, and he regained a sense of control over his health, confident in knowing he was protecting both his heart and his nerves.

Please note that Jeremy's experience is unique to him and does not guarantee similar results for others. Individual results may vary, and it's essential to consult with a healthcare professional to determine the best course of treatment for your specific situation.

If you're among the millions of Americans taking a statin medication to lower cholesterol, it's time for a frank conversation about what that choice means for your health, especially if you're also battling neuropathy.

For decades, we've been told that high cholesterol is the enemy, and lowering it by any means necessary is the goal. But emerging research is changing that narrative. It's becoming clear that the relationship between cholesterol, statins, and overall health is far more complex than we've been led to believe.

This discussion is particularly important for individuals with neuropathy. Studies have revealed a concerning link between statin use and an increased risk of developing neuropathy or making existing symptoms worse. Sadly, many patients and even some physicians aren't fully aware of this potential side effect. This chapter is about empowering you with the information you need to weigh your options and advocate for your own health.

Statin Side Effects: The Hidden Costs

Let's take a closer look at how statins lower cholesterol and the potential downsides of this approach.

- **Targeting Your Liver:** Think of your liver as your body's cholesterol production center. Statins work by essentially hitting the brakes on this process. At first glance, this seems like a solution to high cholesterol, but there's a catch...

- **The CoQ10 Connection:** Your liver doesn't just produce cholesterol. It also creates a vital substance called CoQ10. Imagine CoQ10 as the gasoline that powers your cells, particularly your muscles and nerves. Unfortunately, statins interfere with the production of both cholesterol AND CoQ10.

- **The Nerve Impact:** Your nerves are energy guzzlers. When statins deplete their CoQ10 fuel source, it can cause nerve dysfunction, leading to weakness, pain, fatigue – the very symptoms associated with neuropathy.

- **Beyond Neuropathy:** Statins have been linked to a wide range of issues beyond nerve problems. Common complaints include muscle aches, brain fog, blood sugar imbalances, and even increased risk for diseases like Parkinson's and liver damage. While some dismiss these risks, they significantly impact your quality of life, especially when layered on top of neuropathy.

Understanding Statin Risks: What the Science Says

The research paints a concerning picture: there's a clear link between statin use and neuropathy that many patients and even some doctors aren't fully aware of. Understanding this risk is vital when making informed choices about your treatment.

Who's Most at Risk?

Certain factors increase your likelihood of experiencing statin-induced neuropathy:

- **Existing Conditions:** Those with diabetes or neuropathy before starting statins are at higher risk of worsening symptoms.
- **Age:** Our bodies process medications differently as we age, increasing the chance of side effects.
- **Medication Mix:** Drug interactions between statins and certain medications can worsen the problem.
- **Vitamin D Deficiency:** Low vitamin D levels

might make nerve damage from statins more severe.

The Misdiagnosis Trap

Imagine this troubling scenario: you begin taking a statin, and your neuropathy gradually worsens – increased burning, weakness, and difficulty walking. Often, this is assumed to be disease progression, leading to:

- **Increased Dose:** The logic may be flawed, but it's common to think "more medication" equals better cholesterol control. Unfortunately, this can backfire with worse side effects.
- **Unnecessary Medications:** Doctors might focus on covering up your nerve pain instead of searching for the root cause.
- **Undue Stress:** Believing your neuropathy is worsening compounds the physical and emotional burdens you're already facing.

Delayed Recognition

Sometimes, people with statin-induced neuropathy actually improve initially as their cholesterol falls.

However, this honeymoon period fades as the longer-term damage sets in.

Key Takeaway: If you are on a statin, ANY change in neuropathy symptoms – for better or worse – deserves serious consideration. It's crucial to discuss these changes with your doctor rather than assuming it's simply your disease progressing.

The Power of Informed Choice

Deciding whether or not to use statins is a complex issue. Your doctor should carefully assess your cardiovascular risks alongside the potential for serious neuropathy complications. This is a discussion about what kind of life you want to live, and your voice is vital throughout the process.

Protect Your Heart, Protect Your Nerves

There's great news for those concerned about heart health: protecting yourself doesn't have to mean a lifetime of medications like statins. Natural strategies offer a powerful way to support your cardiovascular system while also addressing the underlying factors that worsen neuropathy.

Looking Beyond Cholesterol

Imagine inflammation as a wildfire raging within your blood vessels. Over time, this causes damage, making them rough and inviting cholesterol buildup. This is the perfect environment for dangerous plaque formation, increasing the risk of heart attack or stroke. While statins temporarily mask high cholesterol, they don't put out the fire of inflammation.

Oxidative damage is another culprit. Think of your cells as constantly creating "exhaust" as they generate energy. Antioxidants act as your body's internal air purifier. However, lifestyle choices and chronic inflammation can overwhelm this system, causing your blood vessels to essentially "rust" from within.

Why This Matters for Neuropathy

Your nerves are incredibly vulnerable to both inflammation and oxidative damage. The same factors harming your heart also worsen nerve dysfunction. By addressing these root causes, you protect your entire body, especially those sensitive nerves.

Lifestyle: Your Most Potent Medicine

Let's talk about the incredible power of lifestyle changes to safeguard both your heart and nerves. The foundation is a diet built around whole, unprocessed foods. Think of those vibrant fruits and vegetables as an antioxidant army! It's also critical to manage your blood sugar, as spikes inflict widespread damage, especially to your nerves.

Movement matters too! Even with the limitations of neuropathy, find activities that work for you. Gentle exercise boosts circulation (vital for nerve health) and helps calm inflammation.

Finally, stress reduction is essential. Stress hormones are major players in heart disease and nerve dysfunction. Mindful practices, even for a few minutes daily, can have a profound impact.

Supplements: Targeted Support

While a healthy lifestyle is your foundation, specific supplements can offer additional support:

- **Omega-3s:** Found in fish oil, these are inflammation-fighting superstars benefiting both heart and nerves.
- **Blood Sugar Heroes:** Magnesium and alpha-lipoic acid help keep blood sugar stable, preventing damaging spikes.
- **Antioxidant Powerhouses:** Resveratrol,

turmeric, and many others offer unique protection against oxidative stress.

Important Note: Supplements work best alongside healthy habits. Talk to your doctor before starting any, especially if you take other medications.

Taking Charge of Your Health: Navigating Statin Choices

This chapter isn't about creating fear around statins. It's about ensuring you have the necessary understanding to make the best possible choices for your unique situation. Whether you're taking statins currently or considering starting, let's explore how to navigate this decision thoughtfully.

Partnership, Not Passivity

If you're on statins, it's important to consult with your doctor before stopping abruptly. A supervised plan may be needed. Instead of being a passive recipient of care, become an active partner in managing your health.

Questions for Collaboration

Here are questions to raise at your next appointment:

- "What are my specific cardiovascular risks? How does this statin help address them?"
- "Could lifestyle changes potentially reduce my need for medication?"
- "Are there any side effects I should be watching for that may signal a problem with this statin?"
- "Could we explore non-statin cholesterol management options?"

A Comprehensive Approach

In some cases, statins may be a necessary piece of the puzzle. However, the RESTORE approach emphasizes a holistic strategy. By addressing inflammation, blood sugar balance, and other key factors, you'll protect your heart, minimize potential statin side effects, and safeguard your nerves.

Knowledge is Power

Understanding how statins work, their potential risks, and the power of natural alternatives empowers you to take charge of your health. It's not about fear-mongering; it's about making choices based on the best available information.

True Health is the Goal

Our focus isn't just on lowering a cholesterol number. True health means healthy nerves, a strong heart, and feeling your best. This often requires a strategic combination of lifestyle shifts, targeted supplements, and carefully considered medications when needed.

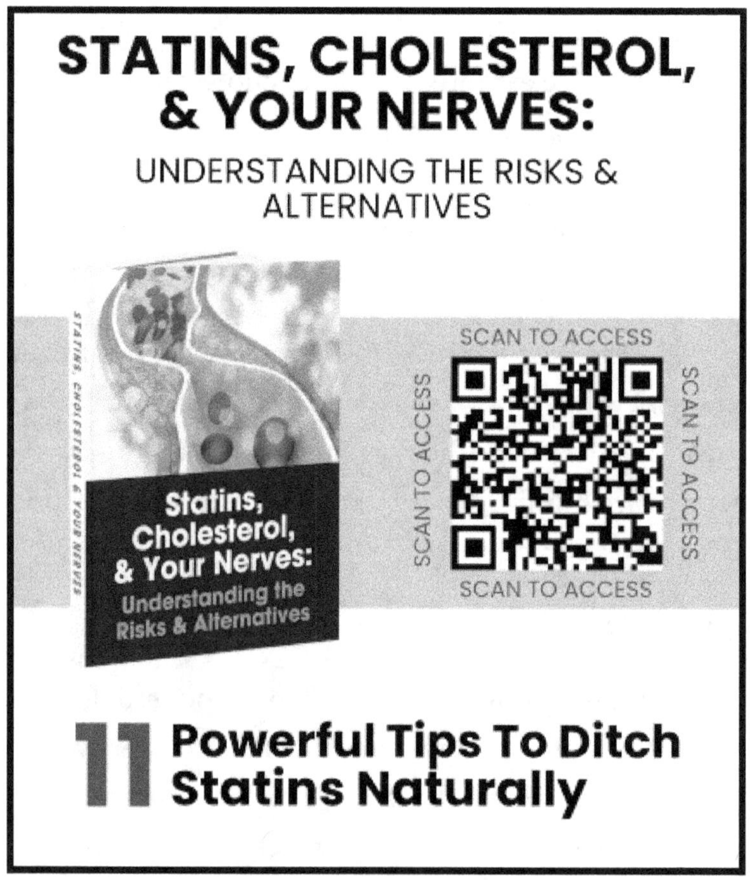

Unlock Your Path to Neuropathy Relief Now: Dial (239) 374-8654 to Speak With Us Today!

10

___

THE GLUTEN-NEUROPATHY CONNECTION: UNMASKING A HIDDEN CULPRIT

Susan came to me at her wit's end. For years, she'd been battling a constellation of seemingly unrelated symptoms: debilitating fatigue, brain fog, recurring joint pain, and a stubborn tingling sensation in her hands that made it difficult to knit, a beloved hobby. She'd seen numerous specialists, undergone countless tests, but received no clear answers. "They keep telling me it's all in my head," she said, her voice laced with frustration.

As I listened to Susan's story, a familiar pattern emerged. Her symptoms, while diverse, pointed towards a possible culprit: gluten sensitivity. While she didn't have full-blown Celiac disease, her body was clearly reacting negatively to this common protein found in wheat, barley, and rye. Gluten sensitivity can trigger widespread inflammation, which wreaks havoc on the nervous system, often manifesting in a variety of seemingly unrelated symptoms.

We decided to try an elimination diet, meticulously removing all gluten from Susan's diet for several weeks. The results were remarkable. Her energy soared, the brain fog lifted, her joint pain subsided, and even the tingling in her hands significantly diminished. By addressing this hidden trigger, we were able to calm the internal fire of inflammation and give her nervous system a chance to heal.

It's important to note that Susan's experience is unique to her. Eliminating gluten may not produce the same results for everyone, and individual responses to dietary changes can vary.

Susan's experience highlights a crucial point: sometimes, the key to unlocking better health lies in looking beyond conventional diagnoses and considering the impact of seemingly innocuous dietary components like gluten.

Let's delve into the world of gluten, a protein found in wheat, barley, and rye, and explore how it might be influencing your neuropathy. This is a topic worth investigating, as understanding gluten's potential impact could be a major step forward in your health journey.

Gluten Everywhere

It's important to realize that our modern diets are loaded with gluten. It's hidden in processed foods, sauces, and even some medications. This constant exposure can be problematic, especially if you have an underlying sensitivity.

The Gluten Debate

There's no denying the controversy surrounding gluten. Some dismiss concerns as a fad, while others recognize a link between gluten and various health issues, including neuropathy. While gluten may not affect everyone the same way, growing research suggests a potential connection to nerve damage that shouldn't be overlooked.

Beyond Celiac

Remember, you don't need full-blown celiac disease to be affected by gluten. Sensitivity exists on a spectrum. Even milder cases can create widespread inflammation, and your nerves are incredibly vulnerable to this damage.

Understanding Gluten: Friend or Foe?

Let's demystify gluten and understand why it causes trouble for some individuals. It's important to note that gluten itself isn't inherently bad. It's a protein found in grains like wheat, barley, and rye. The problem lies in our modern, gluten-rich diets and how certain bodies react to it.

The Problem with Digestion

For those with sensitivities, gluten doesn't break down properly. Imagine it like sticky burrs clinging to the delicate lining of your intestines, causing irritation and damage. This leads to "leaky gut," where things that shouldn't slip out – like toxins and undigested food – start circulating in your bloodstream.

Why Nerves Suffer

Picture your nerves as delicate communication wires. Imagine a fire raging around those wires. Inflammation is that fire, and your nerves are incredibly sensitive to its destructive effects.

Leaky gut is like pouring gasoline on the fire. It triggers a cascade of immune responses, flooding your body with inflammatory chemicals. This constant state of high alert puts immense stress on your nerves.

Think of inflammation as having two damaging effects. First, it directly irritates and injures your nerves, causing those uncomfortable neuropathy sensations. Secondly, ongoing inflammation disrupts the repair and maintenance mechanisms that normally keep your nerves healthy. It's like trying to fix a leaky roof in the middle of a hurricane.

Molecular Mimicry: A Case of Mistaken Identity

Think of your immune system as vigilant security guards with a "most wanted" list. Molecular mimicry occurs when a substance resembles a known threat, even if slightly different. Gluten, for those with sensitivity, can look enough like nerve tissue to confuse the system.

This resemblance, combined with inflammation from leaky gut, can trigger a tragic misunderstanding. Your immune system, in a misguided attempt to protect you, may start attacking both the gluten and your own healthy nerves.

A Vicious Cycle

This mistaken attack further fuels inflammation, which fuels the attack... it's a devastating cycle that can dramatically worsen neuropathy. This highlights why lowering inflammation is key for nerve health and why identifying triggers like gluten is so important.

Gluten & Your Nerves: Unraveling the Link

We've explored how gluten triggers inflammation, but let's make this more concrete. How does this specifically affect your neuropathy?

Imagine your nerves as delicate electrical wires. Inflammation creates chaos. It irritates nerves, causing pain, tingling, and those misfiring signals characteristic of neuropathy. Worse, inflammation blocks your body's natural repair processes, making it hard for damaged nerves to heal.

Warning Signs & Symptom Overlap

Gluten's impact extends far beyond just gut problems. Here are some potential signs that it's contributing to your overall health challenges and making your neuropathy worse:

- **Digestive Distress:** Bloating, gas, and changes in bowel habits are common red flags that your gut is unhappy.
- **Brain Fog:** If you struggle with fatigue, poor concentration, or mood swings, the brain-gut connection is worth considering.

- **Aches & Pains:** Systemic inflammation can manifest as unexplained muscle or joint pain.
- **Skin Issues:** Eczema, rashes, and other skin problems often reflect underlying inflammation which can be traced back to your gut.

It's important to remember that everyone reacts to gluten differently. For some, eliminating it can have a dramatic impact on their neuropathy. For others, it might be just one piece of a broader healing plan.

Is Gluten the Culprit? Finding Answers

Unfortunately, diagnosing gluten sensitivity isn't always straightforward. Let's explore why your test results might not tell the whole story and discuss how to get clearer answers.

The Limitations of Celiac Testing

Standard celiac tests look for a specific set of antibodies in your blood. A positive result is a strong indication of celiac disease. However, your immune system can react to gluten in subtler ways that don't always show up on these tests. This means you could still be experiencing negative effects, even with a "negative" test result.

Your Body Knows Best

Ultimately, your body's own response is the most reliable indicator. This is where a carefully conducted elimination diet becomes your best investigative tool.

The Gold Standard: Elimination Diet

Here's how it works:

- **Complete Removal:** For at least 3-4 weeks, you meticulously eliminate all gluten from your diet. This means being a vigilant label reader!
- **Track Your Progress:** Notice improvements not only in your neuropathy symptoms but in digestion, energy levels, and overall well-being.
- **Reintroduction:** Methodically reintroduce gluten and closely monitor how you feel. A noticeable worsening of symptoms is a clear sign that gluten is a problem for you.

Going Gluten-Free: What to Consider

While the benefits can be significant, it's important to be prepared for a few challenges:

- **Nutritional Balance:** Gluten-free alternatives to bread and pasta aren't health foods. Focus on naturally gluten-free options like fruits, vegetables, legumes, and alternative grains for vital nutrients.
- **Social Adjustments:** Navigating meals away from home requires planning and clear communication. Finding a support network makes this transition much smoother.
- **It's One Piece:** Gluten may be a significant trigger, but it's rarely the only factor in neuropathy. The RESTORE approach addresses blood sugar, inflammation, and nerve regeneration for the most comprehensive healing.

Think of a gluten-free diet as removing a major roadblock. It sets the stage for your body's natural healing abilities, combined with the RESTORE program, to work most effectively.

The RESTORE Difference: Amplifying Your Progress

Going gluten-free, when necessary, is a powerful step towards better health. But remember, even if it's a major trigger, healing is a process. This is where the RESTORE approach shines.

- **Addressing Existing Damage:** Even when the cause of inflammation is removed, your nerves may need extra help to fully regenerate. RESTORE therapies directly target nerve repair, increase circulation, and soothe lingering inflammation for optimal recovery.
- **Tackling Other Root Causes:** Your body is complex. While gluten might be a major culprit, there may be other factors driving inflammation – like blood sugar issues, stress, or nutrient deficiencies. The RESTORE program is uniquely designed to address these underlying contributors for lasting results.
- **The Power of Combined Strategies:** Think of going gluten-free as removing a barrier to healing. RESTORE therapies then actively accelerate the rebuilding process. Together, they create a powerful synergy for true nerve recovery.

Understanding gluten's potential impact empowers you, regardless of how heavily it's affecting you. This knowledge lets you make informed dietary choices that support your health journey.

By addressing gluten sensitivities and utilizing the multi-pronged RESTORE approach, you create the ideal environment for lasting neuropathy relief. This is where true hope lies – not just in managing symptoms, but in achieving lasting transformation.

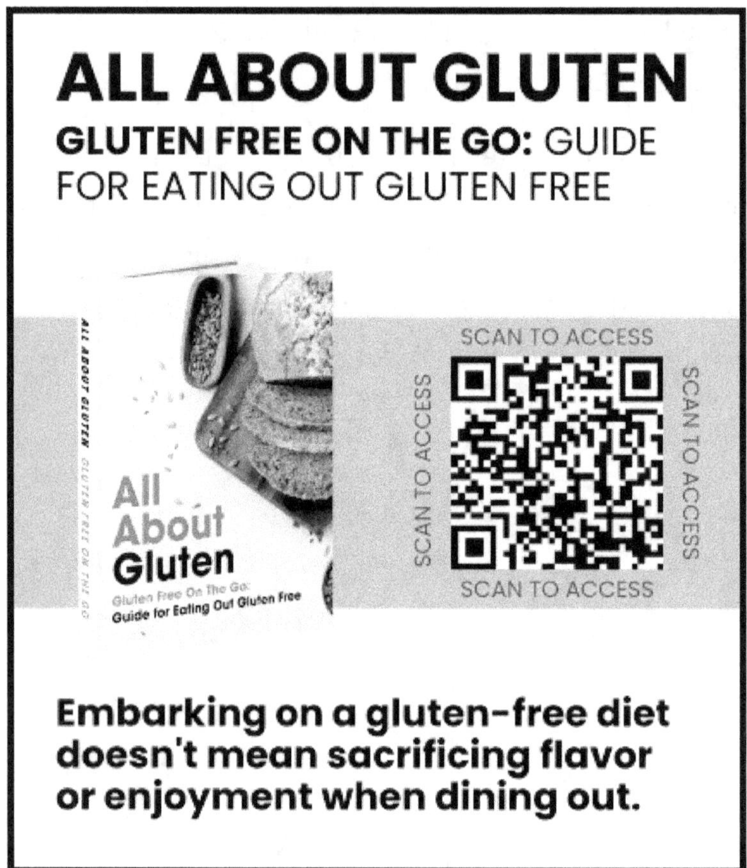

Unlock Your Path to Neuropathy Relief Now: Dial (239) 374-8654 to Speak With Us Today!

11

SCIENCE-BACKED STRATEGIES TO SUPPORT HEALING

"It's like my legs are constantly buzzing, even when I'm just sitting still," Mark lamented, a look of exhaustion etched on his face. He'd been living with painful diabetic neuropathy for years, the burning and tingling sensations making sleep elusive and daily activities a struggle. Medications provided only temporary relief, and he was weary of their side effects. Mark was searching for a solution that addressed not just his symptoms but also supported his body's natural healing capacity.

Knowing that compromised circulation is a major contributor to neuropathy pain, I wanted to explore therapies that went beyond simply masking discomfort. We incorporated Red Light Therapy into

Mark's treatment plan, using specific wavelengths of light to stimulate cellular energy production and promote healing within his damaged nerves. Additionally, we introduced targeted supplementation with L-arginine and L-citrulline, amino acids that enhance the body's production of nitric oxide, a potent vasodilator that improves blood flow.

The combination proved to be a turning point for Mark. Over time, the buzzing in his legs subsided, the burning pain lessened, and he experienced a noticeable improvement in sensation. He was able to sleep better, walk further, and engage in activities he'd long given up on.

While Mark's experience with Red Light Therapy and targeted supplementation is encouraging, it's important to remember that individual results may vary. These therapies may not be suitable for everyone, and it's essential to consult with a healthcare professional to determine the best course of action for your specific condition.

Mark's experience highlights the power of combining natural, science-backed strategies that work synergistically to support the body's remarkable ability to heal and regenerate, even in the face of challenging conditions like neuropathy.

Conquering neuropathy requires a multi-faceted approach. We need to address inflammation, blood sugar, nutrients, and the nerves themselves. This chapter explores three exciting tools that support healing: Red Light Therapy (RLT), L-Arginine, and L-Citrulline. These work with your body's natural processes to promote a healthier environment for nerve regeneration.

Red Light Therapy for Neuropathy

Think of RLT as specialized, healing light. Specific wavelengths of red and near-infrared light stimulate your mitochondria, the cellular power plants. This energy boost allows cells to repair damage, function better, and combat inflammation.

The Science Speaks

Multiple studies support RLT's potential for neuropathy:

- **Reduced Pain & Improved Function:** Research shows RLT can lessen those uncomfortable neuropathy sensations and improve nerve function.
- **Nerve Regeneration:** In lab studies, RLT promoted regrowth of damaged nerves.

- **Diabetic Neuropathy Benefits:** RLT has demonstrated improved blood flow and wound healing for those with diabetes-related neuropathy.

How RLT Helps with Neuropathy

Red Light Therapy offers a unique approach to combating neuropathy by targeting several key factors that hinder healing:

- **Taming Inflammation:** Chronic inflammation is like a fire raging around your nerves. RLT helps to calm this inflammatory response, creating a more conducive environment for your nerves to repair and recover.
- **Boosting Circulation:** Think of your blood as the delivery system for oxygen and essential nutrients your nerves need. RLT stimulates the growth of new blood vessels and improves blood flow to damaged areas, aiding the healing process.
- **Nerve Regeneration:** Perhaps most excitingly, RLT shows promise in directly encouraging the regrowth of damaged nerve fibers. This offers hope for reversing the

underlying damage of neuropathy and achieving lasting improvement.

Practical Considerations

If you're considering Red Light Therapy, here are a few important factors to keep in mind:

- **Options:** You have choices! At-home RLT devices come in various shapes and sizes (pads, handheld devices, etc.). They offer convenience and accessibility. You also have larger, more powerful RLT setups for deeper tissue penetration. Your specific needs and budget will guide the best choice.
- **Consistency is Key:** RLT isn't a one-and-done treatment. For most individuals, seeing significant benefits requires regular use – often several sessions per week over an extended period. Think of it as building blocks; each treatment contributes to a cumulative positive effect.

Remember, RLT is often best combined with other RESTORE strategies for optimal results.

L-Arginine: The Circulation Hero for Your Nerves

Think of L-arginine as a key player in promoting healthy blood flow, especially important for neuropathy. It's an amino acid (a protein building block) found in foods and produced by your body. L-arginine gets converted into nitric oxide, a powerful molecule with a vital job.

Nitric Oxide: Your Blood Flow Superhero

Picture nitric oxide as a master traffic controller for your blood vessels. It signals them to relax and widen. Why does this matter for neuropathy? Think of your nerves, especially those in your feet and hands, as needing a constant supply delivery. L-arginine, by boosting nitric oxide, helps ensure those vital nutrients reach the areas where they're needed most.

Benefits for Your Nerves

We often focus on blood flow when discussing L-arginine and nitric oxide, but they have a profound impact on the nerves themselves through two key ways:

- **Taming the Inflammation Fire:** Chronic inflammation is a major barrier to healing, further damaging your nerves. Nitric oxide acts like a firefighter, calming this harmful inflammation. This creates a better environment for your nerves to repair and recover.

- **The Regeneration Spark:** Some early research suggests that nitric oxide may directly encourage the regrowth of damaged nerves. Imagine it as not only delivering supplies for repair but actively supporting the rebuilding process. This offers hope for reversing the underlying damage of neuropathy and achieving lasting change.

Dosage & Considerations

Here are a few things to keep in mind if you're considering boosting your L-arginine:

- **Food Sources:** While foods rich in L-arginine are beneficial, a targeted supplement may be needed for significant neuropathy support.
- **Dosage is Key:** The right dosage is individual. Work with your doctor to determine the best amount for your specific needs, especially if you take other medications.

- **Safety First:** Discuss L-arginine with your doctor before starting. They'll ensure it's safe for you and monitor its interaction with any existing medications.

L-Arginine's Secret Weapon: Meet L-Citrulline

L-citrulline is an often-overlooked amino acid that works behind the scenes to boost your neuropathy-fighting power. Found in foods like watermelon, it shines brightest as a supplement due to its unique way of increasing your nitric oxide levels.

The Nitric Oxide Shortcut

Think of L-citrulline as taking a clever detour to boost your nitric oxide levels. When you take L-arginine directly, some of it gets broken down during digestion. It's like your body sees it as suspicious and detains it before it can do its job.

L-citrulline, on the other hand, is much better at slipping past unnoticed. This means more of it reaches your bloodstream intact. Once absorbed, your body efficiently converts it into L-arginine, leading to a greater boost in nitric oxide production and all the benefits it brings.

Why L-Citrulline Outperforms

Think of your digestive system as a series of security checkpoints. When you take an L-arginine supplement, some of those amino acids get flagged and broken down before they can reach your bloodstream. This means only a portion of your supplement actually provides benefits.

L-citrulline, however, has a special passkey. It's better at evading those digestive defenses, meaning more of it gets absorbed into your blood. Once there, your body efficiently converts it into L-arginine. It's like sneaking in a larger supply of resources, ultimately giving you a more potent boost in nitric oxide and all those nerve-healing benefits.

Benefits for Your Nerves

Since L-citrulline effectively ramps up L-arginine production, its benefits for neuropathy mirror those discussed earlier:

- **Improved Circulation:** Healthy blood flow is crucial for delivering those nutrients your nerves crave for repair.
- **Reduced Pain:** By increasing blood flow and calming inflammation, L-citrulline may help ease neuropathy discomfort.
- **Regeneration Potential:** Early research hints that L-citrulline may actively support

nerve regrowth. This offers hope for lasting relief.

Dosage & Safety

The right L-citrulline dosage depends on your needs and other medications. It's essential to consult with your doctor to determine the best approach and ensure it's safe for you.

Natural Strategies: A Powerful Combination

The RESTORE approach embraces the power of multiple therapies working together. Red Light Therapy, L-arginine, and L-citrulline create a powerful synergy for combating neuropathy.

A Multi-Pronged Approach

The beauty of combining Red Light Therapy, L-arginine, and L-citrulline lies in their ability to address neuropathy from multiple angles simultaneously. Each therapy targets different aspects of the healing process:

- **Red Light Therapy:** Cellular Repair: This innovative therapy delivers healing light energy to your damaged nerves. This helps reduce inflammation and may directly stimulate the regeneration process, laying the groundwork for recovery.

- **L-Arginine & L-Citrulline**: Boosting Blood Flow: These amino acids enhance your body's production of nitric oxide. This vital molecule signals your blood vessels to relax and widen, improving circulation. Think of it as transforming those congested roads to your nerves into smooth highways, allowing oxygen and essential nutrients to reach areas in need of repair.

Together, they create a healing environment far greater than the sum of their individual benefits. By targeting blood flow, inflammation, and nerve regeneration simultaneously, you set the stage for lasting improvement.

The Natural Advantage

Many conventional neuropathy treatments primarily focus on numbing pain or masking other symptoms. While sometimes necessary for temporary relief, they don't address the underlying damage causing your discomfort. It's like putting a bandage on a leaky pipe – the problem still festers underneath.

Conversely, Red Light Therapy, L-arginine, and L-citrulline support your body's inherent ability to heal. They work with your natural systems to clear inflammation, improve blood flow, and encourage regeneration.

This approach provides a more sustainable path to recovery. You're not relying on medications with a laundry list of potential side effects. Instead, you're empowering your body to rebuild those damaged nerves and restore optimal function, potentially leading to lasting relief from neuropathy.

Important Note: Even natural approaches warrant personalized guidance. Discuss them with your doctor to ensure safety, determine the best dosages, and monitor potential interactions with existing medications.

Red Light Therapy, L-arginine, and L-citrulline work with your body's own capacity to heal. They tackle nerve damage, inflammation, and poor blood flow – the key roadblocks to recovery. They provide an optimal environment for your body to do its remarkable work of repair and regeneration.

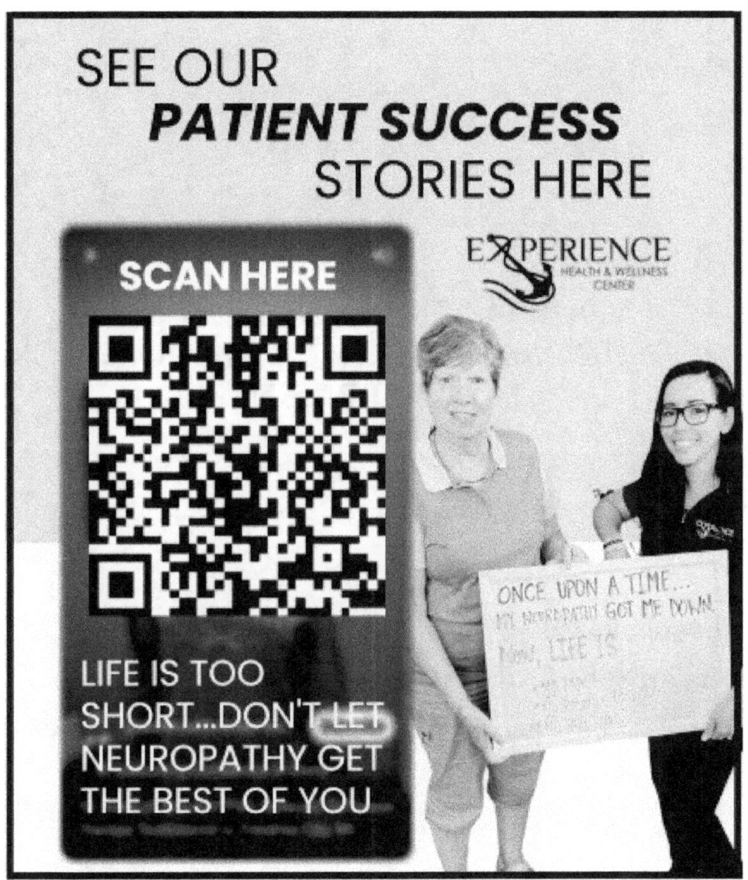

Unlock Your Path to Neuropathy Relief Now: Dial (239) 374-8654 to Speak With Us Today!

12

YOUR FUTURE STARTS NOW: CHOOSE R.E.S.T.O.R.E., CHOOSE EMPOWERMENT

The memory is still vivid. Gail, a vibrant woman in her early 60s, walked into my office with a weariness that went beyond her years. Neuropathy had slowly chipped away at her life, turning simple pleasures into painful trials. She'd tried everything - medications, physical therapy, even acupuncture - but the relief was always fleeting, the side effects often unbearable. The spark in her eyes had dimmed, replaced by a quiet resignation.

But Gail wasn't ready to give up. She was willing to try one more time, this time with a different approach. Together, we embarked on the R.E.S.T.O.R.E. method, starting with a deep dive into the underlying causes of her specific neuropathy. We addressed her blood sugar imbalances, uncovered hidden nutrient deficiencies, and worked on calming the chronic inflammation that was fueling her pain. Week after week, I witnessed the transformation. The pain lessened, the numbness receded, and that spark returned to her eyes, brighter than ever. Gail began walking without her cane, gardening again, and even dancing with her grandkids - activities she thought were lost forever.

It's important to understand that Gail's experience is an individual one and may not be representative of typical results. The R.E.S.T.O.R.E. method is designed to address neuropathy holistically, but individual outcomes can vary depending on a variety of factors.

Seeing Gail reclaim her life is a constant reminder of why I do what I do. It fuels my passion for helping others break free from the limitations of neuropathy and rediscover the joy of living.

Throughout this journey, we've explored the complexities of neuropathy and the limitations of conventional treatment. If you're yearning for a different approach, one that tackles root causes and supports you holistically, the time to act is now. The RESTORE Neuropathy Program offers a pathway towards greater health, reduced suffering, and the chance to reclaim the life neuropathy has tried to steal from you.

This Is Your Moment: Seize the Opportunity for Transformation

Embracing the RESTORE journey means:

- **Investing in Yourself:** This program is a commitment of time, energy, and resources because YOU are worth feeling your absolute best.
- **A Collaborative Partnership:** We work together, your active engagement fueling the success of the personalized treatment plan and support we provide.
- **Hope Rekindled:** Even if past treatments failed, RESTORE's focus on root causes and its multi-faceted approach opens new doors to healing.
- **It's Not About Perfection:** This is a journey of both targeted action AND self-compassion along the way. Setbacks are opportunities for course correction, not signs of failure!

Why Choose RESTORE?

- **Stop Chasing Symptoms, Start Seeking Solutions:** RESTORE gives you a roadmap to WHY your neuropathy is worsening, allowing us to create a truly targeted approach.

- **Less Trial and Error:** Personalized testing and strategies tailored to you reduce frustrating, time-consuming guesswork many patients have endured.
- **Beyond Numbing the Pain:** We prioritize lasting improvement in nerve health, reducing the intensity and frequency of your worst symptoms.
- **Restoring Your Life, Not Just Relieving Distress:** RESTORE empowers you to regain independence, enjoy activities you miss, and thrive despite this chronic, often unpredictable condition.

Your Next Step Starts with One Simple Action

Call us at (239) 374-8654 or visit us at efchealth.com/neuropathy to schedule your neuropathy evaluation. This is your chance to:

- Discuss your unique struggles and goals in a no-pressure setting
- Begin exploring root causes to determine if RESTORE is the right fit
- Learn more about program specifics and how it seamlessly integrates into your life

This evaluation is for informational purposes only and does not constitute a guarantee of specific results. Individual outcomes may vary.

Life with neuropathy can be more than coping—it can be conquering. The tools to change your story, take back control, and thrive are within reach. Choose the R.E.S.T.O.R.E. journey and unlock a future full of possibilities, where neuropathy no longer has the final say.

SCHEDULE YOUR
NEUROPATHY
CONSULTATION HERE
SCAN HERE
SCAN HERE
SCAN HERE
SCAN HERE
EXPERIENCE
HEALTH & WELLNESS
CENTER

9 798889 569955